Prescribing Sunshine

Why vitamin D should be flying off shelves

M. Aziz

Prescribing Sunshine: Why vitamin D should be flying off shelves
First print edition, August 2012

ISBN: 1478396075
ISBN-13: 978-1478396079

Disclaimer

The author will not be held liable for any adverse outcomes that may result from acting upon information in this book. Precedence must always be given to the advice of qualified health professionals.

Audience outside of the United Kingdom: Please note that this book has been written in British English.

Contents

"It is man's consolation that the future is to be a sunrise instead of a sunset." – Victor Hugo

Introduction: D & I

My younger brother cannot talk. He has severe learning difficulties. He is autistic.

Born on a February in the early 1980s, he was lucky to have survived as a premature arrival thanks to one available incubator. Though low in weight with a large head covered in translucent skin, the care provided helped him become a seemingly healthy newborn.

It wasn't until after the age he was supposed to speak that concern grew about his development. I was a late talker, but my brother did not utter anything significant beyond *mama* or *baba* at the same age. A hospital investigation soon confirmed my parents' worst nightmare. Adding to the blow was his diagnosis of knock knees, a condition where both legs turn inward and touch at the caps. This made walking problematic and uncomfortable.

For his autism he was offered speech therapy which yielded no progress. His knock knees persisted, leading to the diagnosis of rickets, a childhood bone softening disorder. It wasn't until his early teens that he was able to have corrective surgery, leaving him with two large scars down the sides of his legs; but this finally allowed him to enjoy walking and running. Prior to this, he was advised soya milk over cow's as doctors believed his rickets may have been caused by an allergy...

As the years passed my brother's behaviour deteriorated. He turned from a boy that engaged in some play with me as a child to one that became self-absorbed and less co-operative. His days at a popular special school were a negative experience too, and he ended up residing entirely at home under the care of our mother.

A few years after he was born she herself began to complain of bodily pains which she attributed to the intense care she had to offer. Unfortunately, it wasn't as simple as that, it was osteoporosis. Her bones were said to be paper-thin. At the time, and even now, it was unheard of for a woman in her mid-thirties to contract this disease. Resultantly, despite drug intervention which helped to prevent fractures, she developed curvature of the spine that chopped down some height. Regardless of her painful condition and the development of further complications such as arthritis and iron-deficiency anaemia she continued caring for my brother.

It became clear that the cause of his rickets and her osteoporosis was *likely* one and the same. Though the link had never been clearly defined I was regardless kept an eye on due to being an at risk candidate.

While I have remained free of bone problems my brother hadn't seen the back of them. Shortly after his operation his legs returned to a slight knock-kneed position. At the time this was believed to be out of habit from his previous state. As it did not impact his ability to walk and he appeared to be in no pain no more was thought of it.

A decade later, however, my brother was unable to get up off the floor. Once leveraged into standing position he could walk, but sitting back on the floor would test my strength in getting him up again. Getting him seen to at A&E didn't help as the doctors focused on treating the thigh rash he developed in reaction to a muscle rub I believed would help him. They believed what resembled herpes was his underlying problem.

The fortunate misfortune was that weeks after he was seen he had two seizures. The result of that was for him to be given long-term what he was prescribed briefly after his legs operation. My brother's diagnosis was the adult form of rickets: osteomalacia. I recognised the given vitamin D and calcium as it formed part of our mother's repeat prescription.

This was the moment a light bulb appeared over my head, albeit dimly. Why was my brother not offered a permanent vitamin D and calcium regimen straight after his legs operation? Since our mother already took both in combined tablets it would have been a no-brainer to consider offering it to him too. The preoperative advice about soya over cow's milk is also unforgivable due to calcium *alongside* vitamin D being implicated in bone maintenance since the early 1920s.

Why did I not raise this issue back in the 1980s? I was just a child myself then and there was little or nothing available to the public to distinguish the sunshine vitamin.

The development of bone diseases in my brother and mother but not myself seemed strange. More so considering that there is no evident history further up in my maternal or even paternal family trees. My maternal aunt, however, did develop severe arthritis, and one thing that links both sisters together is leaving their childhood home of Pakistan for the markedly less sunny England...

Not wanting to take any risks after my brother's diagnosis a doctor advised me to have a vitamin D test myself. It turned out that I too was severely deficient and likely had been for some time. The reason why I may have avoided bone problems could be due to simply treading a fine line or genetic blessings from my father who only suffers general back pain. Whatever the reason, I decided to pop common over-the-counter pills as suggested.

The light bulb above my head flickered a little brightly after a general GP check-up – just months after my vitamin D deficiency diagnosis – revealed I had mildly high cholesterol levels. This did not result in a printout for cholesterol-lowering medication but if my levels remained that way it would've been considered.

While luck may have preserved my bones, my cholesterol reading was unsettling, because the one strong illness link in my maternal family history is indeed heart disease. It had taken my grandfather at a relatively young age, and my mother had developed heart failure just years before my brother's seizures. My father's genes could not provide a safety mat here as he, a long-term sufferer of high blood pressure and cholesterol, went on to develop diabetes in his late sixties. Interestingly though, my paternal family history of health is better than my maternal one; possibly because my poor, dark-skinned father, and those before him, played outside on the abundantly sunny streets of Multan, whereas my comparatively pale mother was often sheltered within a haveli (mansion) in Lahore.

Being inquisitive and living in an era where information literally is at the fingertips, I pondered if the only two things *wrong* in my blood tests were connected in some way. I was surprised to be proved correct, but I thought I must be misinterpreting. At that point I had very little interest in healthcare and knew how easy it could be to link one thing to another by cherry picking.

A part of me, however, could not let it go, so I spilled my

thoughts on the link between cholesterol and vitamin D in a personal blog site entry [http://v.gd/t4gtEZ] in hope that someone would read the post and tell me why I was wrong. Then I could drop the subject and be happy.

I proved unsuccessful.

Not long after I published the piece the Vitamin D Council of America linked it on their news page, resulting in an extraordinary number of hits, elevating the post's ranking in the top search engines for associated keywords. Of the tens of thousands of hits to date not one person has disputed what I theorised. Or should I say what I thought I theorised.

Just a year prior to my post Dr. David Grimes of the Royal Manchester Infirmary created a small ripple in the medical world by questioning if cholesterol-lowering drugs called statins work by mimicking vitamin D. In my opinion this ripple should've been an earthquake, but perhaps the powerful aftershock has yet to arrive.

Enthused by the fact that I shared an opinion with at least one medical professional my blog entry grew in size as I added new findings and shared some familial experiences. I received many comments, one of which was from Dr. Grimes himself who gave the messy piece a thumbs up. As my knowledge grew so did my dissatisfaction with the status quo.

While it is true that doctors were instrumental in diagnosing and treating members of my family, I came to realise that not only were their epiphanies late in the case of my brother, they were also backed up by inadequate treatment guidelines. They have no consensus. Despite attending the same hospital, my brother and mother had different information on what a sufficient level is and how to achieve it.

By fortune my brother's endocrinologist was one of the rare breed of doctors who was more than happy to be flexible on treatment. I explained to him my understanding of vitamin D and presented a short abstract of a study, to which he did not find the need to explain the error of my audacity. Had I presented something outlandish I would have gladly not forced the idea upon the provision of an explanation.

Convinced by everything I learnt I became tired of trying to prove myself wrong. I needed to do something with my fully lit light bulb. This book is that something.

I wrote what you're reading not just for a few people. This problem affects us all. Vitamin D deficiency is a major pandemic and addressing this health concern could result in a radical overhaul of healthcare worldwide. You may find this a bold claim, but if you're willing to read the rest of this book I am sure you will be won over. I can tell you right now that vitamin D is not even a vitamin. It would be more accurate to call it hormone-like. It ranks as highly as food, water and the air we breathe.

To say vitamin D deficiency is connected to almost all ills *is* very audacious. But the truth of the matter is that your body is riddled with vitamin D receptors. You can think of these as solar panels waiting to relay energy to your body parts. The body, however, is very clever and can perform a number of tricks to compensate for deficiency – but only for so long; in the same way auxiliary power in a machine is not meant as a permanent replacement for main power.

Note too that the vitamin D you find in some shops and pharmacies is not the same as what you are able to make through sunlight exposure on the skin. You would also be shocked at the disparity between what's recommended and what nature could give you.

Just as I have observed some pattern of illness in my family it is likely you have too in your own. You may have attributed this to the lifestyles you lead or just bad luck. I believe, however, that what links you and your family's health problems could be the same thing that links me to mine. Why one vitamin D deficient person gets different illnesses to another is largely in the genes.

Of course though, I am not a doctor, so why should you choose this book over one by a white coat? This title, like any of theirs, lets the medical literature do most of the talking, but I add colour by relaying important personal experiences. I show and tell. You will need to trust me. I have adopted a semi-professional voice throughout here but only in order to appear polished, not to impersonate a scientist.

There are parts where I present *theories* by others and myself, but the distinction is made clear. These are important to stimulate debate and to fill in areas where future studies will eventually have the final say.

I'm not shy about appearing as a search engine pundit and I believe I have the gall to say that I know more about vitamin D than many overworked but otherwise knowledgeable and caring healthcare practitioners, who aren't relayed the latest data on the subject. I care because this matters to me. You too will think as I do because this book isn't built on health supplement company press releases but actual scientific papers and review articles. You can look up abstracts and full texts for verification in the references section. Single references per a claim are mostly offered so as not to swell up the book.

I must disclose that due to the immense cost required to read all the papers referenced, a number of sources were selected on the basis of their free summary text (abstract) alone. I defend this practice in that I often cite abstracts with clear, unambiguous statements that should not prove contrary to the full texts. Where feasible, I reference open access articles that are entirely free to the public, thus for that and other reasons it has not always been possible to cite *primary* sources over secondary ones. I leave it up to the reader to thoroughly investigate claims of deep interest; in fact I actively encourage that as you shouldn't just take my word. Could I be wrong somewhere? Yes. Any perception of cherry picking facts would be allowable too as I do not hide my bias towards vitamin D; after all, this book is about selling the subject. However, there has been no intentional dishonesty on my part. My approach may put me under crosshairs and be a disservice to other proponents of vitamin D, but hopefully it is of consolation that I at least care to admit it. If anything, this should help to keep you on your guard. I would like to add that I am not affiliated to any vitamin-related company.

This book doesn't completely blow its own trumpet, though. It acknowledges orthodox arguments on the dangers of the sun and even an opinion that vitamin D is bad for you. If this small portion of the book makes more sense, so be it. But I would hedge that it's because you didn't read from cover to cover, which I strongly recommend.

A handful of interviews conducted in the latter half of 2010 with individuals well-qualified to comment on specific sub-topics feature after relevant chapters to add weight or extra illumination to statements in this book. Responses have been edited for clarity and their inclusion does not necessarily imply mutual endorsement.

If you're thirsty for further commentary upon finishing the book I suggest following my blog at prescsun.com.

News on vitamin D is appearing almost daily so some parts of the book may be behind the times if you're reading this long after its publication.

The ironic thing, then, is that the future of medicine may not be exclusively linked to vaccines and powerful drugs, but to something that has been with us all along.

1. Awakening

From even before the day you're born you need vitamin D.

Pre-eclampsia is a common condition that occurs in pregnant women. It is characterised by various symptoms, the most obvious of which is high blood pressure alongside large amounts of protein in the urine. Left untreated it can cause organ damage and progress to eclampsia – a dangerous but rare condition where seizures develop; foetal development is also compromised.

Research has indicated that vitamin D deficiency can lead to pre-eclampsia.[1] Other theories have been suggested but I believe none are more important.

The reason why pre-eclampsia is a common pregnancy complication in light of this finding is because very few women are vitamin D sufficient. Once a woman becomes pregnant her body not only has to deal with the physical and emotional stress of the situation, her already low vitamin D levels may dip further as the body drives reserves towards an as yet sun-deprived new life. Humans do not thrive with inadequate amounts of vitamin D, so nature will oppose old life when a compromise has to be made. Any infection a vitamin D deficient pregnant woman acquires at this point would certainly be more harmful than usual to her and her child.

Mainstream treatment for pre-eclampsia and eclampsia is magnesium sulphate (a large dose intravenously) to prevent seizures. Magnesium is found in leafy green vegetables, meat and dairy, so it is not necessarily lacking in many diets. However, to aid oral magnesium absorption vitamin D is required.[2] Selenium deficiency has also been implicated in the conditions[3] but it is unlikely to be a more common factor in the developed world where it is not scarce in foods.

First time mothers and those who suffer from illnesses such as heart disease or diabetes are the most likely to suffer from pre-eclampsia. The reason in first timers is due to bodily rejection of the father's genes in a foetus. A mother's body can perceive a threat from what is not genetically hers and mount an attack, but a tolerance can build up for any subsequent pregnancies from the same father due to the adaptive immune system – the part which *learns* how to deal with foreign material – being eventually able to deal with it in a more considered manner. Innate immunity can be seen as the frontline army not prepared to differentiate between approaching friends or foes unless briefed; all must be attacked.

Vitamin D, fortunately, optimises innate immunity[4] which can invoke a ceasefire on certain material straight away. This should theoretically allow people with donated organs to not require immunosuppressive drugs to stave off rejection.

Women who suffer from heart disease, diabetes and other diseases are already immunologically compromised making them more likely to suffer recurrences of pre-eclampsia regardless of adaptation to their partner's genes. If high blood pressure persists after delivery the term pre-eclampsia no longer applies. In many cases the problem resolves by itself, but traditional motherly roles which keep a woman indoors as much as she was during pregnancy will naturally decrease her chances of making vitamin D. Therefore, her blood pressure could remain high because of this.[5] Associated problems such as persistent weight gain could also be linked.

Even if a vitamin D deficient child is born without complication it is not yet out of the woods. If the mother breastfeeds her child, her milk will naturally be lacking in vitamin D unless she deals with her deficiency.[6] Should she opt to provide bottled milk, it may not be fortified with the vitamin depending on what country she is in. Even so, the fortification provided is bound to be inadequate compared to the form and level found in a sufficient mother's milk. But it would be better than nothing. The reason why a baby relies on a mother's store of vitamin D even after birth is perhaps part of a safety mechanism; a newborn is not ready to go out into the open, fend for itself and obtain sunlight.

Things get worse. Even if the child secured enough vitamin D as a baby, once he or she is weaned off their daily source a replacement is harder to find. On top of that, unlike any other animal on Earth, they are clothed and sent to nursery, then school. Incidental sun exposure, therefore, only occurs when travelling to and from these environments – if they are not taken there by transport – or playing outside.

As touched on in the introduction, humans have the ability to create vitamin D when their bare skin receives adequate amounts of UVB radiation, unhindered by pollution or suncream, and when their shadow is shorter than them.[7] If you walk into a darkened room, place your hand against a wall and shine a mobile light on it; – it could be a torch or lit phone screen – you'll notice that the further the light is from the hand, the shorter its shadow. The shorter your body's shadow is outside, the higher the sun is in the sky which is optimal for making vitamin D. If your shadow is too long, the sun is low and in no way over you.

But things aren't easy for the very old who, like autumnal leaves, are destined to fall than prosper. The reason for this is that less cholesterol is sent to elderly skin for conversion into vitamin D. It's nature's cruel but logical way of delivering us to death. However, this does not mean we cannot cheat nature by orally supplementing with vitamin D. Those interested in immortality or at minimum a smoother old age may find this a sort of elixir of life, or at least a component of it. It has been noted that longer telomeres on our chromosomes – think of them as similar to caps on a pen which prevent ink from drying – are associated with longer, healthier living. At least in women, high levels of vitamin D are associated with these not shortening.[8]

The problem with existing vitamin D guidelines is that they are based on a deficient population worldwide. At a top hospital in London, England a normal range for vitamin D – more specifically 25OHD and not 1,25D, as the latter is not indicative of reserves for the whole body – is roughly 20-120 nmol/L (nanomoles per millilitre). Some countries measure this in nanograms per millilitre (ng/mL). To convert nmol/L to ng/mL you need to divide by 2.5; multiply by that to convert in the opposite direction. Our range in other countries then is 8-48 ng/mL.

A conjecture on how this range was produced would be that researchers identified the minimum level needed to be free of rickets or osteomalacia, then sought out persons with the highest levels who perhaps do not supplement and are in good health. It is unlikely that they would have examined the level at which toxicity starts as it would be unethical to do, plus it is not an easy thing to achieve and observe. Those who measured around 120 nmol/L to help create the maximum reference are bound to be young fair-skinned people who thoroughly enjoyed a long sunny holiday or working climate, or perhaps use a tanning bed. Since vitamin D is still currently mostly associated with bone health, for a doctor to be satisfied you only need to reach the 'acceptable' minimum.

To confuse matters, in England there seems to be no definitive reference range. At another popular London hospital I learned the minimum starts from 50 nmol/L (20 ng/mL) while 70 nmol/L (28 ng/mL) is declared most desirable. In that same hospital two different consultants offered contrasting doses, measured in IUs (international units), to my mother and brother. While there is indeed no universal dose it was striking that my brother was and is taking more than her; a difference of 3400 IU. I take more than her too. His osteomalacia has disappeared while she is still osteoporotic, if less than before. That is not to say a higher dose would cure her or repair the damage done. I must confess, however, that I have not seen my mother's vitamin D levels. I cannot intervene for someone who can communicate for themselves and appears satisfied with their treatment.

It is not weak to obey mainstream guidelines, if anything it shows trust and respect for our care providers. The vast majority of their expertise is not to be ignored. But when you're simply not convinced by an orthodox view you will gravitate towards the radical. This applies to anything in life. The latest vitamin D guidelines *will* become mainstream in time though, once they go through all the proper channels. When that is, however, is unknown. The onus is on an individual to treat themselves now or when it may be too late.

When I had my level tested for the first time at the former stated hospital in mid-2006, I measured a mere 10 nmol/L (4 ng/mL). According to recent American guidelines by one laboratory this is severely deficient,[9] and it is unlikely that in 2006 they classed my level as acceptable either. However, my otherwise respected specialist went by our book and suggested an over-the-counter supplement for my 'slight' deficiency. This translated as a recommendation to take the commonly found vitamin D2 at 400 IU. What perplexed me was, had my brother's endocrinologist seen me at his hospital, I would have been offered a much higher prescription-only dose, regardless of being apparently asymptomatic. At the time I did not question the dosage and took a daily gelcap.

The following year I reached 21 nmol/L (8.4 ng/mL). This satisfied my doctor, of course, because I was now 'in range', yet I was still lower than my brother who would not have been allowed to stay at that level. This seemed bizarre. I wondered if I was overreacting and thought maybe vitamin D doesn't matter as much to me as it does to my mother and brother. However, my maternal family history of illness burdened me.

I eventually learned, thanks to the Vitamin D Council through their website [vitamindcouncil.org], that a suggested median dose for beginning repletion is 5000 IU of natural vitamin D3. The target to aim for was 125-200 nmol/L (50-80 ng/mL) which was at odds with both hospitals...

The form of vitamin D didn't bother me but seeing four figures instead of three for the dose made me choke. Though my brother takes large amounts, *I* had not been advised to do that. A study convinced me, however, that vitamin D was safe to experiment with.[10] I therefore decided to give it a go and if I didn't experience any side effects I would continue with it for a year and then get tested. Ordinarily, you should check your level every three to six months, but as an asymptomatic scrounger on the NHS (National Health Service) I allowed myself to be lax. Furthermore, to get a 25OHD test through my GP than a hospital requires a visit to a separate clinic. In-surgery blood drawing would have motivated me more.

The first hurdle, then, was obtaining a high dose of vitamin D. The best I could find in the physical world was 1000 IU at a popular local supplement shop, but the bottle didn't state if it was D2 or D3. Fortunately, from specialist outlets, D3 is very cheap and easy to find at higher doses. The main selling point for D3 over D2 is that it's natural to all animals and it's the form we make on sun exposure. Most importantly it doesn't deflate the wallet.

Taking the capsules with low fat yoghurt to aid absorption turned out to be a non-event. I did not experience anything really positive or negative to my awareness. After a month I was satisfied that I could take this for a little while and not keel over.

Eleven months later my level reached 79 nmol/L (31.6 ng/mL), which in America would be sufficient – but not optimal. I did not tell my specialist I had upped my dose, but as I was not *directly* told to take 400 IU anyway I wasn't technically being disobedient with my foreign over-the-counter purchase. My level did surprise me as I wondered if I would ramp up to 125-150 nmol/L (50-60 ng/mL) and hopefully not much higher. 5000 IU may have been a perfectly acceptable dose for the goal had I not been so deficient to begin with.

The following year I had my blood drawn again after twelve months on 10,000 IU via one 50,000 IU capsule every five days. I reached 141 nmol/L (56.4 ng/mL) which is seen as optimal by the aforementioned American guidelines. However, the hospital reference did not change so I was advised to lower my dose by half. This was an unknowing recommendation of 3000 IU more than they would have allowed.

It was just months after starting the 10,000 IU when I began noticing significant positive changes that I could feel or see in general blood tests. These will be revealed in the coming chapters. Such effects were almost certainly due to reaching a truly ideal level, comparative to those few who get significant amounts of sun exposure as nature intended.

What this proved to me was that while at 79 nmol/L I was no longer deficient, being sufficient was only a marginally better status. To become optimal was to reap the full effects. You can compare being sufficient to eating a starter course at a restaurant: it will sate some of your hunger but you are still hungry. If you want to be truly satisfied nothing less than the main course will do.

2. Skeletal Effects

Ask someone at random what vitamin D is good for and you'll see their brain whir for a second before usually correctly guessing that it helps keeps bones strong. Television advertisements for dairy products fortified with the vitamin explain how calcium products alone are inferior, but vitamin D's effect on bone is just the tip of the iceberg. Nonetheless, our skeletons are the foundation of our bodies.

The unearthing of vitamin D began as a search for the treatment and prevention of bone-softening conditions in children and adults, respectively called rickets – due to bones being seen as rickety – and osteomalacia. These conditions will have been around ever since man decided to wear clothing outside of winter and swapped hunting spears for work under a ceiling.

In 1919 Sir Edward Mellanby found that confined puppies kept away from any source of ultraviolet light developed rickets. Feeding them cod liver oil cured them, leading him to believe that rickets was a dietary concern.[11] Later, Elmer McCollum isolated the magic part of cod liver oil which came to be named vitamin D as it was the next available alphabet letter. The reason it was tagged a vitamin is simple: vitamins are nutrients we consume in order to thrive and this beneficial substance was found in a fat, therefore there could be no dispute.

Harry Goldblatt and Katharine Soames expanded understanding by discovering that sunlight or UV light produced something virtually identical in the skin.[12] An investigation by Alfred Hess and Mildred Weinstock added weight to this by finding that UV-exposed skin fed to lab rats protected them from rickets. The icing on the cake came when Adolf Windaus outlined the structural differences between the plant and animal forms, resulting in the names vitamin D2 and D3.[13] In technical terms they are respectively called ergocalciferol and cholecalciferol. Both words are portmanteaus, highlighting that they are calciferol (vitamin D) derived by other means (ergo), in this case plants, or from animal cholesterol. There is also a D4 and D5 which are analogues of natural vitamin D. Analogues are synthetic copies used as pharmaceutical drugs. The reasons for their development are explained in the chapter *Approaching Repletion*.

It became clear that vitamin D, due to its structure and the fact that it did not have to be ingested, was not actually a vitamin at all but a type of steroid. However, because it had been discovered during a nutritional revolution, to discard it from the fashion would be to lose kudos. Another reason is that moving from the name vitamin D to calciferol would be to lose a more attractive label. Because we correctly think that a balanced diet can provide all the nutrients we need, so do we wrongly believe that the amount of vitamin D we can find in some foods is all that's required.

What about a vitamin D1? Its name suggests that it arose just prior or at least alongside vitamin D2. D1 is D2 with lumisterol, an additional substance that appears on the natural creation of ergocalciferol. To my knowledge D1 has never been used for treatment, perhaps because there is no therapeutic value in retaining lumisterol.

Parathyroid hormone (PTH) and vitamin D play off each other like people on a see-saw. As one goes up the other falls, though you would prefer it if PTH remained closer to the ground.

Parathyroid glands which are found in your neck, and not to be confused with the thyroid glands which they reside behind, produce PTH. These glands are responsible for controlling the amount of blood calcium through this hormone. You need some calcium in the blood in order to live, so if your level falls too low you will die. If it's too high you could also become ill and die. A high level could indicate a tumour in one of the glands causing excessive PTH production, but in most cases PTH elevates when you do not have enough vitamin D. The reason why we have parathyroid glands is simply for backup. As poor summers provide less opportunity for vitamin D production, rather than dying of hypocalcaemia, – the opposite of hypercalcaemia, which is high blood calcium – PTH takes out a 'loan'. But like all loans you're in trouble if you don't pay them back.

The tricks that PTH performs are to steal calcium from the bones to put into the blood, which can be detrimental to the skeleton if persistent, and to increase the amount of *activated* vitamin D – as opposed to the inactive form we can only create or consume for later activation – in the kidneys, which hurriedly absorbs any calcium we ingest. The kidneys also reduce reabsorption of phosphate from our calcium-leached bones to prevent kidney damage.

As supermarket product advertising will tell you, you need vitamin D to effectively absorb calcium just as you need cement to secure bricks on a building. Taking high amounts of calcium on its own can reduce PTH but this is akin to dropping tons of bricks from the sky and hoping enough fall in a fashion to form a vague, ramshackle structure. When you take an adequate amount of vitamin D for your body or expose yourself to ample sunlight, you actually need *less* calcium because it is now being effectively utilised. Unfortunately, mainstream guidance dictates taking more calcium than vitamin D, equating to more bricks than cement and leaving no room for functions beyond calcium maintenance. Why are we dosed in this way? Theoretical vitamin D toxicity. This is also talked about in *Approaching Repletion.*

It may surprise you to know that there is a link between the bone-thinning disease osteoporosis and heart disease.[14] Corroborating this finding is that cholesterol-lowering drugs said to help prevent heart disease have a positive effect on bones.[15] Indeed, one study supported by the maker of the world's best-selling drug of recent times, the statin called atorvastatin, – publicly known as Lipitor[16] – shows that that statin increases vitamin D levels.[17] It is also interesting to note that Lipitor contains calcium. I examine this in depth in the chapter *Cholesterol & Heart Disease,* but in brief what's implied is that it is not high cholesterol which leads to heart disease but the material released from bones that flows into arteries and looks similar to cholesterol. Inflammation is another reason.

Because my brother suffered from bone-softening twice and my mother has osteoporosis, I have been offered precautionary bone mineral density (BMD) scans since my mid-twenties every three to five years. To date I have had two scans. They are quick, painless, and in most cases only the hip and spine need to be scanned. The higher your BMD the less likely your bones are to break.

On my first scan I was relieved to hear that my bone density was fine, this tallied with the fact that I'd never suffered bone pain. At the time I had not been taking any form of vitamin D and was very likely deficient. By the time of my second scan I had been taking 10,000 IU in D3 form which raised me to an optimal level – notably, the only side effect I noticed in the year prior on 5000 IU was frequent non-painful joint clicking which stopped after about six months. I had guessed that my bone density would increase as my PTH had dropped from 4.1 pmol/L (picomoles per litre; hospital reference range: 1.6-6.9) during a vitamin D level of 21 nmol/L (8.4 ng/mL) to 3.7 pmol/L when I had reached a sufficient 76 nmol/L (31.6 ng/mL). It undoubtedly dropped further at 141 nmol/L (56.4 ng/mL) but it was not measured at this point which was when my scan was; in the following two years of increased vitamin D levels, though, my PTH descended to 2.3 then 2.2 pmol/L. The graph below shows a clear downward slope.

Graph 2.1.

My vitamin D and PTH levels over 5 years

(2007-2011, sans 2009)

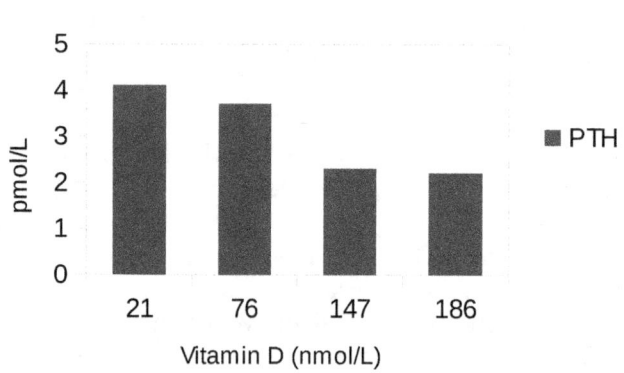

My spinal BMD indeed had risen from 1.076 to 1.156, a 7.4% increase. Additionally, T-scores were provided which compare density to that of a healthy thirty-year-old. In total I rose from -0.6 to 1.0, which are both healthy scores. This was interesting as I was months from turning thirty, the age where you are said to reach the most density you ever will. Z-scores are also used to compare your density to someone your exact age and size, but for me, perhaps due to varying hospital policy, these were not provided. These are also not used to diagnose osteoporosis in older individuals.

In my hip my BMD decreased very slightly from 0.946 to 0.932, yet my T-score rose from -0.6 to -0.7 because of an individual increase in the middle part of my hip (intertrochanteric area). Nevertheless, this was in total counted as a 1.4% decrease, which when viewed on a graph isn't significant. So overall I achieved a 6% improvement in bone density, showing that there was room for improvement since the first scan even though my original readings were normal. If you suffer from common bone and muscle pain or fibromyalgia it is worth seeing what vitamin D could do for you, considering that such sufferers are frequently deficient.[18]

The strange thing, however, was that if my hospital's calcium reference range of 2.15-2.55 mmol/L (millimoles per litre) is correct, my blood calcium was slightly high before vitamin D optimality as well as after. I had measured 2.59 mmol/L in the year before my second bone density scan, then 2.7 mmol/L at the time of it. Neither of these alarmed my doctors because they didn't coincide with other risk factors for hypercalcaemia and the fact that I was asymptomatic. Also, according to one study, hypercalcaemia is defined as a level persistently *above* 2.7 mmol/L,[19] so as far as I know 2.7 is the highest acceptable level, in line with an optimal vitamin D level. Hypercalcaemia could be indicative of excessive calcium release from the bones but that couldn't apply to me with my bone density increase.

The year after the scan though, my unintentionally still optimal vitamin D level of 147 nmol/L (58.8 ng/mL) was accompanied by a better blood calcium level of 2.47 mmol/L. I must add that I took 90 mcg of vitamin K2 MK-7 daily for a season prior to that blood test. I am uncertain if my level would've normalised without it but this is a vitamin that I want to keep as part of my regimen, and it is one that I would advise further personal research on; it has been noted for aiding in bone and heart health. In the following year when I reached a ceiling vitamin D level of 186 nmol/L (74.4 ng/mL) by taking 5000 IU daily for nine months and then 12,500 IU for three months, my calcium *rose* to an allowable 2.52 mmol/L; I had not been taking K2.

A calcium level that falls way at the lower end of the reference range could indicate that the parathyroid glands are making a perilous compromise between satisfying the blood level and bone destruction.

There is no doubt that calcium – and also magnesium,[20] which is overlooked – is an essential component to health. However, it is puzzling that humans are the only animals to consume milk beyond infancy and often that produced by another animal, disregarding cats who do not need it too. Fruit, veg, beans and nuts contain calcium but these are seen as containing inadequate amounts, so we rely on milk and dairy products, not only for their good taste, but to maintain the levels we need. Some also take calcium as a supplement.

But compared to other animals our ratio of calcium to vitamin D seems disproportionate. To recall the brick and cement analogy, why would you need more bricks than your amount of cement could cover? If you lack cement you hope that the weight of extra bricks will compensate.

One study that introduced worry about the use of

calcium and/or vitamin D outlined that intake may be associated with brain injury.[21] The problem with this study was that it was not stated if vitamin D3 – the form natural to humans and other animals – was used. It will have been unlikely due to vitamin D2 being the common prescription. More importantly, the doses used were "approximately equal to the [recommended daily amount] for calcium (mean = 1280 mg) and... lower than current recommendations for vitamin D (mean = 341 IU)." What was not distinguished was whether that amount of calcium – which slightly exceeds common daily intake via food – coupled with an amount of vitamin D that is markedly less than what a naked body could produce daily through UVB attributed to the development of brain lesions. Simply put, they should have tested if high amounts of calcium alone would cause this problem and whether a higher amount of vitamin D3 could be protective. A conjecture on why these brain lesions happened in the elderly is the fact that having less capacity to produce vitamin D in the skin[22] means that they will likely be more deficient than the rest of the population.

The only dairy I consume is a pot of yoghurt or two per day, with total calcium intake from all sources consisting of little more than 500 mg daily. Sometimes I'll treat myself to ice cream, pizza or cheese sandwiches but I don't believe I ever exceed 1000 mg. If you feel your calcium is lacking then a tablet might be wise.

Another calcium product we use is toothpaste which is combined with fluoride to combat and prevent tooth decay. While I do not dispute that regular brushing has helped protect our teeth and gums, there could be a more natural and effective adjuvant than fluoride. I don't need to spell out what that is.

In many developed countries fluoride is also added to drinking water, no doubt as extra protection for people who may be lax in oral hygiene, but there is controversy about its use.[23] Fluoride binds calcium to teeth in a world where vitamin D deficiency is rampant. Given that vitamin D is available in cream form for topical use in skin conditions it would be easy to have it added to toothpaste. Even better than that, you could simply make sure your vitamin D level is optimised, chew calcium-containing foods and brush only with a substance that cleans your teeth and freshens breath.

Sugar has been implicated in causing tooth decay, be it from manufactured or natural foods, as well as acidic food and drink in general. But we do not know if this happens less or not at all in a vitamin D-optimised population. In my teens I used to drink a can of cola every single day; worse was that I had a habit of swilling it around in my mouth before swallowing. Resultantly, on top of likely being severely deficient even then, and despite practising good oral hygiene, I developed some dental erosion. One front tooth lost half its enamel, exposing some dentine. Fortunately, this and no other tooth became sensitive due to halting my fizzy drink intake in time. When I do drink I no longer swill, even with an optimal level of vitamin D. I've kept my dentist happy. It is also wise to remember that carbonated water is not natural. Sugar is fine in controlled amounts, but you need to make sure that your teeth can deal with it in one way or another.

A curious observation in my mother and brother is that despite respectively suffering from bone thinning and softening, neither of them showed signs of expected tooth decay or loss. This particularly surprised the doctors of the former. The local effects of toothpaste with calcium and fluoride must have helped in this area. Had London been part of the 10% of the United Kingdom to have significantly fluoridated tap water[24] it *may* have reduced the severity of their bone conditions, should the level added be enough to have an effect, even if it's not beneficial for us overall.[25] Since water in London is classified as hard it has high calcium and magnesium content,[26] which signifies that neither person had a stark lack of these nutrients to begin with as we consume tap water often.

In a vitamin D deficient population then, the ideal drinking water for the time being would, questionably, appear to be hard and fluoridated. In Wales, where a higher level of dental problems was recorded recently in children than in other parts of the UK,[27] the water is mostly soft and does not have fluoride added to it.[28] Children are also naturally recommended to use pea-size amounts of toothpaste. As noted previously, magnesium must not be overlooked as it is as important as calcium. Some people in the world may be deficient in this if they do not follow a balanced diet; a case where supplementation is essential. Magnesium deficiency, amongst other things, can mistakenly cause PTH to remain low in vitamin D deficiency alongside osteoporosis.[29]

A recent study postulated that depression could lead to the development of osteoporosis. The finding of depressed women having over-reactive immune systems was a correlation.[30] It is true that people diagnosed with osteoporosis can suffer *sadness* for logical reasons, but the onset of depression – which I'll define as distinct from easily attributable sadness – and subsequent low BMD could both be linked to low vitamin D. Seasonal Affective Disorder (SAD), nicknamed "winter blues" for obvious reasons, appears when vitamin D levels commonly reach their nadir.[31] Should this be followed by bone thinning, a vicious cycle then occurs where disability keeps a person permanently housebound which worsens their depression and osteoporosis.

The reason osteoporosis is less common amongst men is due to the additional bone-protective effects of male-level testosterone.[32] Interestingly, a study suggests that this hormone is boosted by higher vitamin D levels in men,[33] at least in those with no underlying testosterone production issues.

Those suffering from a serious bone disorder from birth called osteogenesis imperfecta would also benefit from vitamin D alongside calcium and magnesium due to the likelihood of sufferers acquiring osteoporosis. It may also be true that vitamin D-sufficient mothers protect their offspring from developing the former condition in the womb.

Not all bone disorders are concerned with the breakdown of bone, though. Fibrodysplasia ossificans progressiva turns muscles to bone when damaged, eventually producing a "second skeleton." It is a disordered repair mechanism for which there is currently no good treatment. Vitamin D and calcium are withheld for this condition. Whether vitamin D optimality could treat this disease is unknown to me and it would certainly be risky to trial given how little is known about this rare illness. It is certain, however, that any doses experimented with would have been low. Moving seven letters along, vitamin K may be useful for such sufferers. Found in green leafy vegetables, which are a natural food to most animals, this co-factor *helps* to direct calcium into bone and away from other organs where it can do harm. Some people may be vitamin K deficient which is why a supplement would be useful. K2 is generally seen as preferable over the K1 form but it is slightly harder to find and fairly expensive as a supplement. Complimentary requirements for vitamin D are covered in detail in the chapter *Vegetable, Mineral & Animal.*

3. Brain Development & Maintenance

The term *cognition* refers to the ability to learn and process information. A study found an association between low vitamin D levels and poor cognition in middle-aged to older European men.[34] This finding could be applicable to persons of any age, race or sex. It may also have an impact on how we prevent and treat one particular neurological disorder that arises in infancy.

Dr. John Cannell published a theory implicating vitamin D deficiency as the cause of autism[35] on the Vitamin D Council's website. The non-profit American organisation, in which Cannell serves as executive director, relies on donations to educate the public about the consequences of not being vitamin D replete. Approximately a decade before I discovered his theory the MMR vaccine was being painted as a common culprit. Before a child makes it to nursery they are stamped with this jab to give them antibody-mediated immunity to measles, mumps and rubella.

Anyone who has ever seen the news in the last decade, as of writing, will be familiar with the controversy. Debates were waged everywhere, celebrities voiced their opinions, and uptake of the vaccine dipped, resulting in outbreaks of once curbed illnesses. The doctor at the centre of the storm, Andrew Wakefield, had his original 1998 publication retracted by the esteemed medical journal *The Lancet* in early 2010[36] and this was seen as the final gavel blow on the matter by all but his staunchest supporters.

As the brother of someone with severe autism this theory did very briefly pique my interest. However, I quickly realised that the argument was thin on facts. Yes, rates of autism have been going up but there is only weak circumstantial evidence to blame the vaccine. My brother and I did not even have the combined MMR jab when very young as it was only available five years after his birth in the UK.

When I told a few friends and teachers in primary school about my brother none of them knew what autism was. I knew no one else with an autistic family member, though it is possible, like with myself, that others became less comfortable with talking about a seemingly freak condition. The lauded 1988 movie *Rain Man* appeared when my brother turned five, it was deemed the first piece of work to significantly expose the condition to the mass public. Autism rates, however, began rising remarkably since 1980,[37] in part due to relaxed criteria acknowledging formerly dismissed sufferers. A year later in 1981, Australia introduced the highly successful *Slip! Slop! Slap!* sun awareness campaign[38] that set the template for guidance in other countries around the world.

If MMR can be directly linked to autism and autism spectrum disorders such as Asperger's syndrome, more people should be autistic than there are as the vaccine was given to many children prior to Wakefield's study – regardless of whether it was in the form of single or multiple jabs. Of course, the argument used is that some children are more susceptible to its effects than others, and it's there where the answer may lie. The correct question should be "*if some* children do develop autism because of MMR, why is that?"

The reason the MMR controversy gained such

momentum was because it was dramatic. Usually the first introduction a child has to medicine is the vaccine, so when a child subsequently fails to develop as others do it is logically attractive to accept that the contents of a syringe may be to blame. However, I emphasise, MMR is just one of many things given to young children. As well as vitamin D deficiency through lack of outdoor activity, we often provide them and ourselves with diets that are far removed from what nature intended. To say on the news, for example, that eating rusks could lead to autism would likely meet ridicule. It might be true, but it would not be taken seriously by most because it doesn't sound as grave and places the blame on purchasing-parents.

As a child I suffered from a serious case of German measles (rubella) which hospitalised me for weeks. A huge boil the size of a liberal squirt of ketchup appeared in the crook of my right arm and pus had to be manually drained out of me. Alongside frequent applications of calamine lotion I needed large doses of an antibiotic which triggered eczema on my eyelids that would not shift until my mid-teenage years. This measles struck me despite being vaccinated. However, vaccination did safeguard me from other childhood illnesses. I have not been around anyone with mumps but antibodies to it are ready in my adaptive immune system. Many people think of these illnesses as simply harmless, which is largely true in a vaccinated population; otherwise they can do great harm and even kill.

MMR contains a trio of live viruses which have been modified to be harmless. It does not need to be preserved and, therefore, contains no mercury[39] which has often been implicated as toxic to the brain. There is an argument that there may be too young an age to receive MMR, however, babies are far too young to have to suffer and die from indiscriminate illnesses.

It could be possible that some form of childhood intervention causes autism, but it is also feasible that those who do develop it are vitamin D deficient at root and are resultantly unable to effectively deal with benign entities.

Cannell's theory has some way to go before being proved or disproved, but since the brain requires adequate amounts of vitamin D for normal neurological development and maintenance, and a rise in autism has correlated with compliance to sun safety advice, the case is strong. It certainly fits with my personal view that a deficiency did not cause my brother to only develop rickets and osteomalacia.

Either MMR or other things, possibly in tandem, can cause autism in deficient individuals – for example, the toxin clearing substance called glutathione lacks in such people – or deficiency itself alongside a predisposition is the key factor.

There is also the question of whether the vaccine is needed if it can be proved that vitamin D optimality enables innate immunity enough to fight measles, mumps and rubella effectively. It would explain why the human race did not die out early. But until we know, the vaccine should not be avoided.

A study shows that many autistic people have abnormally low cholesterol levels[40] and that giving them cholesterol supplements ushers improvement in behaviour[41] – likely children whose brains are still developing. This is interesting, but not all autistic people have low cholesterol problems. Indeed, my brother's total cholesterol has measured mildly high which nearly put him on a statin.

You will have heard that some cholesterol is good for you and this is true. In one instance, cholesterol is needed to create vitamin D. Because a large amount of cholesterol can be found in the brain[42] it is assumed it is there for a reason. The brain also contains vitamin D receptors.[43] What this implies is that an inability to create enough cholesterol has the same impact as the ability to create it but not getting enough sunlight to convert it. I would hedge that autistic people with low cholesterol who are supplemented with it show some improvement in their behaviour because, despite still being vitamin D deficient, incidental sun exposure potentially allows them to now create more vitamin D than before.

Autism affects males more than females.[44] One obvious difference between the sexes is the hormone testosterone. Women produce some testosterone but not as much as men; likewise, men do not produce as much oestrogen. Significant oestrogen has been found to protect the brain regardless of vitamin D deficiency[45] whereas testosterone does not.[46] It is interesting to note that women with autism are more likely to have traits such as tomboyism and excessive body hair, indicating higher testosterone levels.[47] To nip Cannell's theory in the bud we perhaps only need to find a male with autism who, at minimum, suffered from testosterone deficiency after sexual differentiation in the womb up until the age of around five-years-old.

What we're seeing here is that protection is key, but what is the trigger of autism? Since vitamin D enhances production of glutathione,[43] it will remove mercury from the body. As pointed out, though, mercury has never been used in MMR. It can be found in some other vaccines in small amounts, but even so it has not been implicated in causing autism, even if doubts remain.[48] Lead is another toxic material we are exposed to in everyday items such as paint or cosmetics that can be passed on to babies.

To pinpoint which toxin is linked to the development of autism, if there is only one, will require further study. Vitamin D, however, should serve whether autism is attributed to brain development itself,[49] toxin removal or both. Because vitamin D deficiency is pandemic it is also likely that genes play a part in susceptibility to a disorder that is no longer rare but not yet affecting all children. There is talk that autistic people are often the offspring of overachieving adults, but this is not true for my brother. I would hedge, though, that many exceptionally intelligent people have high-functioning autism and are not too fond of outdoor recreation, which doesn't bode well for starting a family. Such people may also opt to have children at a later age.

The finding that autistic people are more likely than others to develop rectal prolapse[50] may partly exonerate Andrew Wakefield's belief in there being a shared factor for IBD (inflammatory bowel disease) and autism. My brother suffered from prolapse in his late teens which required surgery. IBD which may lead to prolapse[51] could well be related to vitamin D deficiency,[52] and IBD does not always produce symptoms. One finding that partly supports the toxin hypothesis of brain diseases is a 2010 study which found that 'washing out' a bleeding infant's brain to remove pressure and toxins resulted in less disability.[53]

When my brother suffered bone softening for the second time in his life, in his early twenties, the first symptom he presented was the return of slight knock knees which soon led to an inability to lift himself from the floor. Finally, a seizure before and after his diagnosis of osteomalacia resulted in adequate treatment.

At the time of admission my brother was pre-diagnosed as epileptic. Epilepsy – amongst other problems – is a common finding in autistic people[54] either early or late in their lives, so this seemed logical. But it did not explain my brother's leg problems and the fact that his arms seemed to bruise easily despite care in pulling him up from the floor. Forced to look for something that linked them all together they eventually found him to be severely lacking in vitamin D and calcium. A regimen containing high amounts of both expectantly cured all his symptoms within a season.

A week after he was discharged he suffered his second but final seizure, despite having started treatment. This seizure was thankfully small, indicating a lessening. My brother woke up after half an hour rather than a day or two. As precaution, though, he was referred to a neurologist who dismissed his seizures as being related to anything other than vitamin D deficiency. Five years later he suffered another moderate seizure, but this has been labelled as an isolated event due to running a fever. The fact that he had suffered seizures due to vitamin D deficiency shows that he has acquired a lower threshold than much of the population in relation to many possible stimulants. My mother, for example, did not suffer seizures before or after being diagnosed with osteoporosis.

Had my brother been diagnosed epileptic he would have been offered an anticonvulsant. A form of these drugs are called CCBs (calcium channel blockers). The effect of CCBs on epilepsy is related to their name: they block calcium. If the brain receives more than it requires, perhaps due to excessive loss from bone, seizures can occur.[55] Vitamin D can interfere with the effectiveness of CCBs,[56] perhaps due to competition for its actions. It has not been fully explored if some epilepsy sufferers are simply only vitamin D deficient as they would not be investigated further without presenting bone problems, which can occur later and are then blamed on CCB treatment.[57] However, a pilot study indicates that vitamin D may be taken seriously as an anticonvulsant.[58]

In some cases surgery to remove part of the brain where seizures occur is offered, but preventing calcium from entering is a good first thing to try. As we shall see in the *Cholesterol & Heart Disease* chapter, it is also interesting that anti-cholesterol drugs could stave off seizures.[59]

CCBs are also used to treat depression and bipolar disorder. The difference between the two is that the latter is depression in alternation with manic episodes. A study has shown that in older adults – who are typically housebound – vitamin D deficiency is associated with lower mood.[60] This has implications for all types of mood impairment. Indeed, vitamin D has been suggested as a treatment for both mentioned conditions.[61] You can figure why UV light boxes are touted as beneficial for SAD (seasonal affective disorder). Additionally, the visual presence of sunlight itself can have a positive effect.

Other than mood problems there are other conditions which affect the brain such as Alzheimer's disease, Parkinson's disease, multiple sclerosis, motor neurone disease (amyotrophic lateral sclerosis) and schizophrenia. Each of these conditions has been associated with vitamin D deficiency.[62] [63] [64] [65] [66] Additionally, CCBs have been mooted to have a positive effect on them by study or logic.[67] [68] [69] [70] [71] Alzheimer's disease has also been linked to high cholesterol.[72]

Why I didn't develop autism could be down to luck. One other plausible reason is that I was born just two or three years after my mother migrated from Pakistan to England, and before her outdoor exposure had diminished. Though Pakistan is a Muslim country with a conservative dress code, my mother never engaged in full-body covering or the headscarf which allowed for some reasonable exposure in a sun-blessed country. England has often been characterised as grey and dismal in the weather department but there are frequent surprises, and without any children yet to worry about, my mother was free to enjoy the outdoors as she pleased.

After I was born she adopted the traditional housewife role; looking after the flat and her new child. When I was old enough and the weekend weather was good, she would kit me out in a t-shirt and shorts and took me to local parks. Early 1980s summers were rarely disappointing.

I soon became fit for nursery when the stork was about to deliver again. Early.

For the first few years of my brother's life he appeared normal, his response to our parents and myself was satisfactory. He had been born six to seven years after my mother arrived from Pakistan and several years after her outdoor exposure had severely minimised. I do not, therefore, believe it was a coincidence that she developed osteoporosis and associated conditions a handful of years after giving birth to an autistic son with rickets. She had suffered from depression too that will have been worsened by her vitamin D deficiency.

My brother's golden years, neurologically, may have come about only from depleting our mother's desperate vitamin D reserves while in the womb. British milk is still not fortified with it.[73]

I, on the other hand, was enjoying outdoor play in nursery and the rest of my school life. I would not have been making much vitamin D due to my light brown skin colour and the regular lack of UVB in England, but I would have been making something, while my housebound mother and brother – whose behaviour limited his outdoor exposure – were not. At home we did not consume much foods that contained some vitamin D. The only relevant condition I suffered from, now thought to be linked to vitamin D deficiency directly on the skin, was antibiotic-induced eyelid eczema.[74] My brother additionally suffers from asthma since childhood, and this too is thought to be related to vitamin D deficiency.[75]

Interview: Oliver Gillie

Oliver Gillie is behind the United Kingdom's Health Research Forum, a non-profit organisation dedicated to accelerating the latest scientific data into public health policy. He holds a BSc and PhD in genetics and developmental biology from The University of Edinburgh, and his writings have featured in The Sunday Times *and* The Independent *newspapers.*

What ignited your interest in vitamin D?
Well, I was doing some research on schizophrenia in the early 2000s and I found a lot of research into the genetics of it, with one group saying that it's an inherited disease. Now, there's a lot of problems with the evidence for that, and I thought there's got to be some sort of environmental factor here, and one of the few clues in the literature at the time supporting that was that birthdays of schizophrenics tended to group in the spring or early summer. I then looked for other diseases where this might be the case and I found that multiple sclerosis was another example.

This got me thinking about a cause and I first considered folic acid deficiency before someone suggested vitamin D deficiency. It hadn't occurred to me to look at that as everybody equates vitamin D with bones, – that's the story that we all know about – so I looked at vitamin D and I found that that might indeed explain the birthday findings in schizophrenia and multiple sclerosis.

I then went about finding out what other diseases were

associated with insufficient vitamin D and discovered that some evidence existed for type 1 diabetes, as well as all the bone diseases, of course. There was also some evidence about cancer through the work of the Garlands (Frank [late] and Cedric, USA). This made me think that if it's true that vitamin D is the key cause here, – and if the Garlands' have found a relationship between cancer and latitude – there ought to be a relationship with altitude too because the amount of UVB [to create vitamin D] reaching the Earth varies with height above sea level. So I searched through the literature and found that someone had looked at the relationship because they'd expected that there would be more cancer at higher altitude since you're exposed to more cosmic rays, and it's known that cosmic radiation can cause mutations. But they found the opposite – that there was less cancer, which is what you'd predict from vitamin D being involved.

I then wondered what else could be involved and thought of skin colour. The data on that suggests all sorts of things, but if you look at people with dark skin in the US where the data came from there was more risk of cancer.

So I thought there was something in the cancer story, but these were observational findings, not experimental findings. I was impressed by them though, because in looking at it in three entirely different ways there seemed to be a link and I hadn't expected that. From then on I started following the story very closely and I put together my first book about it [*Sunlight Robbery: Health benefits of sunlight are denied by current public health policy in the UK*] as I was convinced that sunlight was important and we were getting the wrong message about it.

What is your opinion of Cancer Research UK's

conservative sun exposure guidelines?
CRUK – although they deny it – had a total sun avoidance policy at that time. They said that you should put on suncream twenty minutes before you go out, wear clothing that covers your arms completely, wear a hat, and not go out in the sun in the middle of the day. If you follow all that you'd make no vitamin D at all and you'd make yourself quite ill in the long-term, so I think it was very bad advice. Now they say something slightly different: they recognise that vitamin D *might* be important, but it's just a slightly watered down version of the same advice. They say you only need a few minutes of the sun to make enough vitamin D but that's wrong, you need quite a long time.

How much success do you think the Health Research Forum has had in promoting the benefits of vitamin D to healthcare providers and policy makers?
It's been an uphill struggle but the message is beginning to take off now. I think I have actually been quite successful as there's small groups in various parts of the world who have been convinced, and we're all in touch with each other and help each other out, so a lot more people are beginning to get to know about vitamin D.

But there's still many doctors who don't know about it, including cancer ones. A patient might be taking vitamin D because they read about it and think it might be a good idea to optimise their level, but the cancer doctors say you shouldn't be taking anything other than what they tell you. So we've got a long way to go still before the medical profession gets the message; they're beginning to get it and there are some doctors who are quite enthusiastic about it, but they're the exception.

Why can't we find physiological doses of vitamin D in

UK high streets?
Boots the chemist, for example, are very conservative. They completely follow the established maximum levels that are recommended. They won't change that. They're just extremely conservative [and that's the example most other retailers seem to follow].

What's your opinion on the value of vaccination programmes if we become a vitamin D-optimal population?
Vaccinations are a completely separate issue from vitamin D. If you're talking about flu, I think we should have the flu vaccination. Taking vitamin D might help to overcome some of the effects of a flu attack, but I don't know if it'll actually prevent an attack.

How much money do you think the NHS could save if the government revised their policy on vitamin D?
This has been calculated and is in one of my papers; it's about twenty-six billion a year. In Europe as a whole it's around three-hundred billion a year. But that isn't money you necessarily get in your pocket, that's the money the government gets. If somebody has MS and they're in a wheelchair for twenty years it's the family that has the loss of earnings and the cost of dealing with all that, so the savings would be spread out all over the place.

Do you think the burqa – which is optional Muslim dress code – should be banned in light of it exacerbating vitamin D deficiency?
I think the burqa is a health hazard here, there's no doubt about that. Muslims living traditionally in their countries of origin would have houses built around courtyards and the women would be able to sun within the privacy of their home, but that's not possible for Muslims living in

modern flats or houses in Arab or European countries. So I think there is a health problem. However, I don't think that it's practical or sensible to tell people they can't wear a certain item of clothing and if they walk the streets you're going to rip it off them or imprison them. It's a question of sharing what we know.

In one of your publications you mention that rickets affects Scottish and northern English sheep lacking vitamin D. Do deficient animals equate to poor quality meat?
I don't know if the meat's poor quality but it is interesting that sheep are affected. These animals were imported from the Middle East and they've been bred to have very thick coats, so the sun has a lot of difficulty getting through to their skin to produce vitamin D. I therefore believe it's quite important that sheep are sheared at the beginning of the summer. But that's just one of a number of things that can hinder vitamin D synthesis. If they grow fast during the winter when their vitamin D levels are low they can get rickets. If it's a mild winter and the grass is growing and they're feeding well but they're not making enough vitamin D, they can still get rickets. So it's all very complicated but it's all to do with the sheep having a heavy coat.

Should health authorities develop better ties with supplement companies or can pharmaceutical companies be trusted to deliver cost-effective products based on natural vitamin D?
The trouble is that vitamin D can't be patented so it's difficult for [drug companies to get enthusiastic about it]. Anybody could make a product with vitamin D in it, but it also costs a lot of money to get it passed by the MHRA (Medicines and Healthcare products Regulatory Agency).

Do you think Dr. John Cannell of the Vitamin D Council states a good case that autism may be linked to vitamin D deficiency?
It may well be that that is the case but the evidence for that is minimal really. Autistic people are more likely to be born in the late spring or early summer, so it fits in with the pattern of other nervous system diseases such as multiple sclerosis and schizophrenia, and that's a link which I consider to be quite important. But most other people wouldn't attach the same importance.

Have you heard of the Marshall Protocol, which advises against vitamin D supplementation, and, if so, what's your opinion of it?
I do know about that and I have discussed it with some people who've thought about it quite carefully and deeply, and they believe it's just a theory at the moment. There isn't any really strong evidence for it. But I'm a scientist and a writer and when it comes to some judgements about evidence I feel it all gets a bit too complicated for me because there are certain things I don't feel confident about judging. I tried reading about it and I thought there could be something in it, but people with more clinical knowledge than me – as I'm not a medical doctor – felt that this was just a theory with no backup there.

You can visit the Health Research Forum at healthresearchforum.org.uk

4. Vegetable, Mineral & Animal

If you haven't heard of the Paleolithic diet, you're sure to have heard of the Atkins which it's similar to. The Atkins Diet encourages people to limit their intake of carbohydrates such as bread, cereals or sugars, but not their consumption of natural fat. It must be noted, however, that Dr. Robert Atkins did not encourage excessive fat consumption[76] nor rule out a gradual increase of some "carbs" at a later date when an individual is satisfied with their weight, contrary to some media reportage. The popularity of this nutritional approach peaked in the early Noughties.

The Paleolithic diet is not essentially aimed at weight loss, but like the Atkins it promotes a limitation of man-made foods, e.g. bread and cereals. It advocates natural animal fats and fruit and vegetables. The principle of the idea is that we should be eating as man from the Paleolithic era did, as the food found in nature is the food we are meant to eat. It's what's good for us. The Paleolithic era, simply, was when we developed the tools to hunt, fish and cultivate. Both diets have their detractors – and I admit I do not follow either of them – but they have a logic in accordance with vitamin D. Where we once enjoyed regular sun exposure on naked skin, we also did not have supermarkets to purchase unnatural foods from.

For vitamin D to work properly additional factors have to be looked at. This may mean tweaking your diet if you already engage in a balanced one or, as a last resort, considering extra supplementation. Most people, though, don't want to wake in the morning and swallow numerous capsules to start their day, so where possible you should address your nutrition through varied food.

Before you think, then, that you must not take vitamin D pills because it's meant to be made in the skin, remember that it is a thing you can glean a bit from food. Inuits consume vast amounts of *fatty* fish like salmon and tuna, thereby getting more vitamin D than in a common, once daily, over-the-counter capsule. Interestingly, these people have not evolved white skin which, logically, would be advantageous in a sun-deprived climate. I explain why this may be in the following chapter.

Examine foods in a supermarket aisle and you'll find that many are labelled 'suitable for coeliacs'. Coeliac disease is a syndrome where a person experiences a number of symptoms stereotypically related to the bowels in response to gluten in wheat. It can be debilitating. A general wheat allergy produces non-specific symptoms such as breathing difficulties. The fact that such labelling is common indicates two things: that it's no longer a rare condition and that having no such guidance makes sufferers lives a misery.

In some quarters wheat is not even advised for those seemingly able to tolerate it.[77] Some people may not even be aware that they are gluten intolerant because they present no evident symptoms.[78] This suggests that the problem could be more widespread and that, contrary to advertisements, wheat may not be good for you. Absorption can also become impaired in coeliac sufferers which means supplementing with vitamin D would be like putting water in a holed bucket. Should coeliac disease be much more common than we think, wheat avoidance or reduction would be as essential as vitamin D repletion.

I must confess, though, that I do not walk the talk here. As someone seemingly tolerant to gluten I have not been moved to avoid such foods. I also assume it would be as hard as quitting smoking due to how common such items are. Furthermore, I do not find difficulty in maintaining my calcium or vitamin D levels. But I remain open minded.

In recent years vitamin K has also been getting attention. As much as wheat avoidance is part of the Paleolithic diet, so is inclusion of foods containing vitamin K. If you are not lying to yourself and *truly* have a balanced diet, then you shouldn't be deficient in this as it is found in green vegetables, typically of the leafed variety. Nobody disputes that vegetables are natural, but some will have a preference for organic produce. The key benefit of vitamin K is that it helps control blood clotting and drives calcium to the bones.[79] Vitamin D aids in absorption, not direction. Our bodies convert vitamin K1 into K2. There are suggestions, though, that supplementation of K2 itself in a form known as MK-7 may yield better results[80] than relying on limited bodily conversion.[81] Since foods containing K2 are scarce there may be factors which prevent sufficient conversion of common K1.

I am sure many people are not generally vitamin K deficient, so the decision to supplement with K2 MK-7 should be down to personal examination of more evidence elsewhere.

The key thing to remember, though, is having a balanced diet. Paleolithic man would not be downing bowls of pasta regularly; in fact not at all. His food wouldn't ever come in a packet. And he wouldn't be shopping online, away from the sun.

Another thing to avoid – but not entirely – is vitamin A. Seventeen experts jointly authored a review condemning supplementation of this.[82] They reported that vitamin A toxicity, which thwarts the actions of vitamin D, was a common finding in developed countries. In Third World countries, where all-round nutrition is lacking, supplementation had a positive effect. A common source of high vitamin A is cod liver oil. Though it may contain some vitamin D, no one really eats a cod's liver. It is not a natural food. Paleolithic persons would not touch it. I would not worry about the small amounts of vitamin A in natural foods, but I would not supplement with it. The review presents a persuasive argument.

Leading on from this, you may have found some vitamin D supplements combined with vitamin A. When I was first advised to take vitamin D I was informed by a pharmacist – wrongly – that it could only come with calcium or vitamin A. Having had no calcium deficiency I went for the latter. My gelcaps contained 400 IU of vitamin D and 4000 IU of vitamin A. I stopped taking this within a year, solely because I came to realise that the amount of vitamin D was inadequate. I did not know until later the added benefit of stopping this particular supplement. Funnily enough, just a few years later, I began to see vitamin D & K combinations take precedence on pharmacy shelves – around about the time the joint review was released.

Fish oil, which is derived from the body, is fine as we do eat fish bodies. One needs to only look at appraisals for omega-3 fatty acids to see that fish oil capsules may be a worthy investment. But dosing would be important. The amount of fish Inuits typically consume should dictate how much should be in a capsule, or perhaps it should match that of the "proven" American prescription fish oil called Lovaza – marketed in the UK and Europe as Omacor – which is designed to reduce high triglycerides that contribute towards our cholesterol profile. It would undoubtedly be cheaper to take six British triple-strength omega-3 capsules over four Lovaza ones for the same levels of fatty acids. Unfairly, Lovaza's website once compared its four as equivalent to fourteen standard-strength fish oil capsules.[83] Fourteen capsules of anything per day would make anyone baulk at the assumed total price and the chore of having to swallow so many large items.

As much as eating poorly is bad for us, so is a sedentary indoor lifestyle. This combination can be connected to rising levels of obesity in the UK and the existing epidemic in America. One study of many has found that obesity leads to vitamin D insufficiency because the substance gets trapped in excess fat, whether it's produced by sunlight or taken as a supplement.[84] It is probably this more than increased body fat itself which leads to a higher risk of heart disease and other illnesses; particularly in obese males, as females appear to retain protection through oestrogen.[85]

Because vitamin D is converted in the liver, anything that damages the liver can also impair the conversion process. Alcohol is thought to be carcinogenic to the liver – that is, it may cause cancer. Certainly, alcoholism can lead to liver damage and subsequent failure as seen in the well-publicised case of late legendary footballer George Best. Since the liver is the place where vitamin D conversion initially occurs it is perhaps the worst organ of all to get affected and may part explain why significant liver disease is unquestionably fatal.

By adhering to some, or preferably all of these suggestions and other common sense ideas, you allow vitamin D to do its job unimpeded and minimise the risk of side effects. For example, long-term higher than recommended intake has been linked to the formation of kidney stones.[86] Indeed, my brother's endocrinologist warned of this too. However, neither myself nor my brother have developed them in six years of taking 5-12,500 IU. Nor has my mother who has taken 1600 IU for over two decades. This might well be due to following a South Asian diet which, despite some probable faults, comprises a lot of healthy and natural ingredients. Remember too that kidney stones are common in general in a worldwide population that is deficient.

Do other animals require sunshine? Indeed they do. Anything with a spinal column will obviously need calcium to support it[87] and, therefore, vitamin D to absorb it.

Vitamin D expert Dr. Michael Holick wrote in a review that pet iguanas develop osteomalacia or osteoporosis when deprived of sunlight and calcium-rich foods.[88] They are just like us. A BBC News story in 2009 reported that three Sumatran tiger cubs born in Paignton Zoo in Devon, England developed osteoporosis because "a lack of calcium from their mother may be to blame."[89] While this would be true, the zoo did not speculate that an additional factor was their climate. A fourth tiger "seems unaffected." Because furred or feathered animal skins aren't directly exposed to sunlight, such creatures must lick off created vitamin D during grooming for it to get inside their bodies.[90] In essence, their pill bottle is their coat. What's happening to the tigers is a tragedy as these animals are in danger of extinction and could be better served in native conservation programmes.

Some vitamin D can also remain above human skin which is why people are advised not to shower immediately after sun exposure. The reason why this is so could be to serve as a direct healing agent, like antiseptic cream, or because in some cases it takes time to enter the body.

Something that piqued my interest was the discovery that dogs evolved in the Middle East. These smaller descendants of wolves came about through gene mutations in something called IGF-1 (insulin-like growth factor 1).[91] IGF-1's action, as its name suggests, is to promote growth. Its amount rises as vitamin D levels go up, to a certain point.[92] If an animal moves to a place where there is less sunlight, it would be advantageous to produce smaller offspring over a number of generations so that the reduced UVB and subsequent vitamin D production is perfectly enough. The vitamin D and IGF-1 parity would facilitate this. The origins of the domestic cat have also been traced to the Middle East.[93] One need only look at a world map to see that it's just a few steps out of the more sun-blessed Africa, and perhaps the point where we allowed cats and dogs into our homes.

Feather or fur colour doesn't always act as a light filter like skin colour does, which is why humans may only evolve to be shorter when skin lightening alone isn't enough in sun-deprived areas. This might explain the stereotype of many pale Scandinavians being tall; maybe they differentiate from other fair-toned people by perhaps having an adequate vitamin D status[94] thanks to their love of fish – which contains vitamin D. Yet of course, Scandinavians are not the only people to grow tall and other reasons can be involved. Tallness, though, like obesity, can be a disadvantage in a world where vitamin D deficiency is the norm as such people are less likely to *get by* on low levels than those of average or short height.[95] This would be true for horses only rarely allowed to venture outdoors.

But smaller height doesn't help when you can't get any sunlight. Just like tigers can get ill, so can domestic pets who are kept away from UVB. Diabetes in cats and dogs has often been blamed on a sedentary lifestyle,[96] the same as in humans. Pets that don't go out to play are also not getting window-uninhibited sunlight on their fur, – windows block UVB – nor are they getting vitamin D from the livers of prey, and they may not find it in useful amounts in their tinned food. Interestingly, when I visited Pakistan I noticed that domestic cats were taller than ones from the British Isles. Introduced back to sunnier climes, they may have got nature's 'go ahead' to grow again somewhat. They are also not too commonly kept as pets there. Cats though, despite their love of sunbeams, appear to rely more on vitamin D from prey than synthesis due to limited fur cholesterol.[97] They surely must have evolved that way.

Going back to colour, a recent Finnish study has found that brown tawny owls are appearing more often than grey ones due to a warming climate. In cooler climes brown feathers are associated with a weak immune system and it presents poor ability to hide from predators.[98] Though these are nocturnal animals, they rest in sunlight during the day. Animals without feather or fur can be prone to sunburn just like humans and I wouldn't be surprised if this often occurs in those mostly confined or exported from hot to cold climates where UVB is a struggle to acquire.

In a later chapter I explain how vitamin D prevents diabetes in humans. The same would apply to other animals.

There is one other thing than skin colour or mass that helps or hinders vitamin D and that is, as discussed previously, age. Elderly people have a reduced amount of the substance in their skin that is needed to make vitamin D.[22] This could simply be nature's way of programming us and other animals to get ill and die; that we've had our life and that it's time to make way for the new. Though controversial to say, life didn't design for the elderly to live out their extended years in a nursing home. But that doesn't mean elderly people should sit at home waiting to die, they can just take supplements. While young people can create optimal amounts of vitamin D through sunlight, there is no way an elderly person can sustain desirable levels without buying a bottle of pills and getting regular blood tests. This would apply to other animals too.

Another thing that leads on from this is fertility. You may have heard the term "survival of the fittest", so who else would be fittest than those replete with multi-beneficial vitamin D?[99] This leads to the question then, particularly for humans, whether infertility in potentially treatable cases is better dealt with through vitamin D than standard fertility treatments. IVF (in vitro fertilisation) leads to a high rate of stillbirths[100] and birth deformities.[101] If nature is telling you you cannot have children, this should be something to heed.

As this chapter's title suggests, plants also require vitamin D to thrive. They need soil nutrients just as we need food, as well as water, air and sunshine.[102] We happily seat our plants outside or near open windows, but we ourselves won't go out without clothes and sometimes apply suncream. Deprive a plant of food and water and it will certainly die, deprive it of sunlight and you'll see that the plant may bend and produce leaves of lower quality: a slow death. I witnessed this happen to a friend's plant. Remember also that a common form of vitamin D supplement is derived from plants and fungus.

Hemp seed oil is receiving attention for abilities such as reducing inflammation of the skin as seen in eczema[103] or psoriasis. One explanation for this seems to be that hemp seed oil contains the fourth alphabet letter vitamin, at least according to online shops I've visited. Cannabis itself, of which hemp comes from, has been used to alleviate some symptoms of multiple sclerosis.[104]

You should now realise that virtually all creatures and plants that live for the day do so for that very reason: to live. Night-living moles and bats hardly need any vitamin D to stay healthy,[105] [106] but I'm assuming no vampires are reading to ape them.

It is possible that humans could evolve to not need vitamin D if the pandemic remains unaddressed, but this would require unnecessary suffering over hundreds or thousands of years to occur first.

As you can see it's all common sense: live naturally, eat naturally, and you just *might* not need medicines.

5. Human D-volution

Vitamin D deficiency is a worldwide pandemic.[107] Why? Multiple barriers to sufficient sun exposure.

We can safely assume that if there's a large yellow ball shining in the sky it is meant to be there. Also, if nature wanted our skin covered we would've been born that way. Humans are the only living beings on this planet that hide their natural outer layer with material from other animals. Very few people disobey this rule.

The primary reason for the emergence of clothes would be to keep humans warm in cold weather as we could not rely on a decreased amount of body hair compared to our ape ancestors. Over time, clothing would have evolved from basic designs to cater for warmer seasons, general fashion, heightening attraction and tribe differentiation. The end result is that to be seen in public without clothing is embarrassing and disgusting because we are no longer used to seeing too much of each others bodies outside of intimate relationships. Worshipping the sun as a deity also lost favour with the advent of, mainly, the Abrahamic religions.

As it is unlikely that any time soon the majority of humans will adopt naturism, – and that includes myself – the only trade-off for getting adequate sunshine would be to cover up just the private parts when the weather is right and enjoy a day sunning in the park or at the beach. Unfortunately, nine-to-five living and lack of optimal weather in many countries means most people cannot do this frequently. Those who can – and enjoy it – may find sunbathing to be counterproductive if they apply UVB-blocking suncream as advised on the bottle, or enjoy the heat only in the shade of a parasol. Sunbeds that primarily emit UVA should be avoided as their use or abuse has been linked to skin cancer.[108]

Because we're constantly exposing scant skin to UVB light it's easy to see why we have a deficiency pandemic. But clothes are not the only barrier to vitamin D production.

There was a time when working was waking up to search or hunt for food under the gaze of the sun in little or no clothing. Compare this to today where many of us take transport to the confines of four walls and a roof. Save for those who enjoy a packed lunch in the park, most have virtually no significant sunlight exposure during the week. People go home when it gets dark, and again possibly by car, bus or train. That leaves the weekend. Some people will enjoy the outdoors regularly or sporadically when the weather is right, but many would take this opportunity to enjoy indoor activities like going to the cinema or eating out. Others, understandably, use the time to stay at home and rest.

Children have it slightly better. Morning school breaks and lunchtimes are a chance to have fun in the playground, and sports lessons sometimes enforce appropriate under-dressing for an outdoor activity. On weekends and some evenings boys, typically, would go out and play football with their friends on the street.

I say *would* because such happenings are becoming rare. Over the last few decades the leather football has been demoted by a virtual one which can be controlled on-screen with thumbs. The lure of video games is hard to fight. As a child of the 1980s, the decade where home console titles began challenging leisure centre arcade and pinball machines, it was not hard to stay indoors and shun friends. And if I did need them, they would join me in such games. By the mid-1990s it was not even requisite to have all your friends under one roof thanks to online gaming.

Video games differ from traditional board games, construction toys and other forms of indoor entertainment in that you do not bore of them as quickly, and their multitude of 'levels' help to keep you glued to the controller. Modern games consoles solve the physical inactivity part of playing by encouraging you to run on the spot or use a controller as a tennis racket, for example, but these games are still played indoors only.

Another reason why children play indoors more often is because they are not encouraged outdoors as much. We hear on the news, with increasing frequency, horror stories of paedophiles moving into neighbourhoods, kidnappings and street violence leading to death. Whether these crimes have actually increased more than decades ago, it's certain that access to multiple news sources has now rammed awareness of these dangers into public consciousness. While these parental worries are warranted, the likelihood of succumbing to a vitamin D deficiency-related illness is certainly higher than being subjected to abuse.

For children and young adults who have more relaxed parents there is still the dilemma of where to go. When I was growing up there was always easy access to at least a swing, slide and a climbing frame – be it at school or many local parks. As the years passed though, these began to disappear. This can be attributed to the popularity of home computers and videos games, but more importantly the rise of compensation culture.

Over the last decade we have been bombarded with advertisements that ask if you have "had an accident that wasn't your fault" and promising "no win, no fee" for claims made. Such an awareness has instilled a disproportionate fear of getting sued because of how easy the process has become, and how widespread it is.[109] Therefore it's become cost-effective for councils to simply remove playground equipment. Many years before this children and parents accepted the risk from such apparatus and held faith in safety mats and supervision. Children sometimes got hurt, but in most cases the damage would have been less than the consequences of being wrapped in mental cotton wool.

With little or no local equipment small children have less reason to go out and play. The only mercy comes at school break times when they have to improvise something together in their blank playgrounds. For young adults the mass closure of youth clubs – at least as I witnessed in my own area – cemented the excuse for some to not bother going out on weekend days. Others like myself also have obligations to stay at home and look after ill family members. A further portion even contribute to the crimes which fuel parental worries.

Making matters worse is the fact that much of the food we eat lacks vitamin D. In England the only commonly fortified foods are breakfast cereal and some dairy products, yet the amount is still insignificant to have any impact beyond basic bone maintenance. Everyday natural foods such as fish and eggs fare no better unless we eat them in bigger portions and regularly. Aside from this our diets have changed to include a lot of foods that don't aid vitamin D in its job, and those which do *may* be stripped of their benefits to some degree if not produced organically.[110]

Cholesterol deficiency is another factor since we cannot make vitamin D without it. In a previous chapter I explained how cholesterol deficiency could lead to autism in children. Later on I outline how conscious or unconscious cholesterol reduction later in life can impact our health.

A final factor as to why some of us are more deficient than others is migration. In the previous chapter I reasoned how the climate led to the development of osteoporosis in Sumatran tigers at an English zoo. These animals are not indigenous to the country, nor are humans without white skin.

Before you worry that this is turning into far-right propaganda, you must remember that I am brown-skinned. Though I am British by birth, people of my look and colour are obviously native to South Asia; in the same way that white Americans or Australians are native to upper Europe or Russia. If people get exasperated at my answer of London when I'm asked where I'm from, it is understandable. We do not yet live in a highly mixed world and it is in our nature to probe what appears exotic.

The problem is not with migration per se, but migration without adaptation. If man was meant to fly he would've been given wings, if woman was meant to drive she would've been given wheels. This is not to mock transportation as I value vehicles, but we are the only creatures on this planet not often satisfied with just using what nature has given us.

Before high-speed transportation the only way to migrate would be to set off barefoot or on a large animal. To begin with, the only migration would've been out of Africa as that is where humanity originated.[111] We would have had little or no clothes and no map to consult to know where to go and how far. With no itinerary we simply choose a direction, follow it through or take detours, and just settle at places we like. Humans would've made incremental steps further away from the equator as their offspring tired of a place or found territorial competition.

There should be no surprise, then, to see why skin colour evolved as humans moved to less sunnier climes. As a child I was led to believe that skin colour evolved in relation to heat, but what purpose would light skin have in repelling heat – as dark colours draw it in – when the climate is cold? There is a study, though, which suggests a *random* gene mutation resulted in decreased skin pigmentation,[112] and this is corroborated by a suggestion that the appearance of blue eyes is merely cosmetic.[113] I personally find it interesting that both these features are common in cold-climate Europeans who I believe have these traits thanks to their ancestors having adapted to their environment through many generations. Anthropologist Nina Jablonski certainly believes that paleness is an advantageous *intended* evolution in a place lacking UVB as the default protection offered by dark skin – and perhaps eyes – could lead to ill health there.[114] Northern Europeans also appear to have bigger eyes to let more light in, and larger brains due to greater visual processing needs.[115]

One thing that is common to people of all colours is pale palms and soles with not much range in pigmentation. The reason this might be is because these body areas frequently do not face the sun. The soles of your feet do not see the light of day. Even when you're lying down your soles do not face the sun. Likewise, the natural position of our hands is with our fingers curled and palms facing away from the sky. Armpits would be universally pale were it not for the fact that resting our hands behind our head is a fairly natural position. Though parts of our bodies are covered with varying amounts of hair, humans in sun-deprived climates often have brown, blonde or red hair to allow ease of UVB penetration.

But not all "indigenous" communities in cold locations have developed light features. A thorn here is the Arctic Inuit who has black hair and brown skin. Their abundant source of food is fish and they avail of it in high amounts, compared to Americans who could be used as a general benchmark for the Western diet.[116] Fish, of course, contain vitamin D which at a regular high intake is as beneficial as regular sun exposure or high dose supplements. Therefore there is no need for Inuits to evolve pale features as long as this diet is kept up through generations. So it seems low reserves of vitamin D in a family line are the trigger for relative skin lightening. Alternatively, Inuits have not been there long enough for white features to develop yet. The reason Inuits are not black is because their ancestors would have needed to drop a shade in the journey to their end destination. Early groups of Africans would not have sailed directly to the upper north.

A study found that Inuits who have migrated to Denmark often have higher blood pressure than those from near-Arctic Greenland. This has been attributed to the "modern Western way of life", which I believe covers diet change.[117] As far as I know there are no indigenous pale-skinned humans in sunny countries, though I have seen Afghans with green eyes and natural blonde hair. This could be the result of adaptation in progress because of conservative Muslim dress code decreasing UVB exposure; I am just speculating.

Some white and mixed-race people have freckles.

These are pigment-filled gatherings of a light brown colour that can be found in some or many parts of the body. I would confidently hazard that the development – or remainder – of these is a small form of extra protection during sunny seasons in cold climates, or indeed for those who have migrated to hot countries like Australia. Freckles also become more prominent under sunlight. In myself, one tiny dark brown birthmark on my arm could possibly be a resurfaced remnant of my distant African ancestry.

One story from 2003 that grabbed my attention was that of a black woman being born to white Dutch settlers in South Africa. Her grandparents and great grandparents are also white.[118] This certainly isn't a common occurrence which is why it was newsworthy. The only reason I can think of for this 'defect' is that it was perhaps absolutely necessary for her to be black. Why? I cannot fathom. I would be interested in seeing if there are white children born to black parents in colder climates – discounting cases of albinism which is often a complete absence of protective bodily pigment.

It is possible that some such skin colour surprises are just a random happening with no value, such as if an outdoor-loving black couple produced a white child in a sunny country. I am unaware of any such cases but there are mixed-race couples – where both partners are dark-skinned – who have twins with entirely opposite skin, hair and eye colour. One such couple is from England.[119]

What I'm about to explain now could be used against young people if misread, and that is the issue of crime.

Many sociological reasons have been attributed to why youngsters turn to crime, and while issues such as family instability and poverty have rightly been picked up on, the biological side, I feel, has been neglected, either because it's not thought to have as much weight or could be seen as prejudicial. However, to ignore biological factors is a great injustice.

In England it seems as if disruptive behaviour beginning from youth age has increased in recent years, but part of this could be down to better reporting from news media, thus creating an illusion of things getting worse. For instance, a recent England and Wales Home Office report on crime shows a general reduction in recorded incidents during the Noughties;[120] though, of course, victims might be reporting less. But we are aware that crime happens, and whether things have really got worse since years and decades past, we are definitely more wary than we once were. So how does this relate to vitamin D?

The chapter *Brain Development & Maintenance* points out that vitamin D appears essential for growing and ageing brains to prevent problems such as autism or Alzheimer's disease. It also reports that the female hormone oestrogen is brain protective while testosterone is not. This is an important thing to note as most crimes, particularly violent ones, are stereotypically carried out by men.

Prof. Simon Baron-Cohen developed the theory that autism is the result of having an "extreme male brain" where systematising takes precedence over empathy.[121] Not all autistic people are aggressive but many brain disorders, including autism, are linked to aggression.[122] Therefore, with reservation, I believe that men who consistently lack empathy for potential victims are perhaps mildly autistic. Some such people may have found school life too much of a challenge, and later imprisonment doesn't help much either. English data, moreover, shows that at least between 1995-2008 girls have consistently outperformed boys academically.[123] Stereotypically, girls too are less likely to be engaged in crime if you go by what you hear on the news.

A report by The Institute for Fiscal Studies suggests that the autumn-born tend to perform better academically than their summer-born peers[124] which in turn affects employment prospects. While there would be many valid exceptions to this observation, there is one glaring explanation here: the summer-born are carried in the womb during the months where the mother cannot synthesise much vitamin D from the sun. And newborns are rarely taken outside until at least around sixth months.

Poverty can also play a role in vitamin D deficiency as poor parents would be less inclined to add supplements to a diet when trying to make ends meet. Deprived areas also tend to be northern where there is less UVB exposure.

As vitamin D deficiency is rife, crimes related to lack of empathy would present more from males of all races. In the media, however, we can see the dark-skinned monopolise the headlines for negative reasons. Racism can undoubtedly distort the truth, but if there is a propensity for dark-skinned individuals – and this includes myself – to be less empathetic, the answer could in part be due to vitamin D levels below those of whites due to increased natural sun protection.

It is important to stress that it is not only dark-skinned individuals who *could* lack empathy, just that they might be more likely to than whites in climates not providing enough light. The only way to confirm if this is true is to see what all the differences are between high and low-achieving men, be they dark or pale, from across many countries.

One advantage that blacks have over the brown and

white-skinned is higher bone density[125] despite lower levels of vitamin D.[126] Though I have not seen many osteoporosis cases, the only people I know to suffer from it are my mother and another person's white grandmother. The reason blacks possess this advantage could be an evolutionary backup.

Even in climates friendly to black people, season change ushers in less usable sunlight, so it would not be favourable to suffer so easily from a lack of calcium in the blood and bones. Brown and white-skinned people likely lost or never acquired this backup because their level of pigmentation makes it inessential. That does not mean, however, that black people can ignore vitamin D. Calcium absorption is only one benefit, and deficient blacks still suffer from other illnesses related to a lack of vitamin D; in fact probably more so in countries with healthcare inequalities.

Speaking of inequalities, because black people have better bone density, in some sports, the stereotype of them being better athletes then holds some truth. Of course though, not all black people are physically fit and many sports also require being mentally skilful. In aggressive sports, such as boxing, if you pitted a vitamin D deficient white or brown fighter against a black opponent, and both had equal vital statistics and experience, the edge *would certainly* go to the latter; but may even out if both have long-term optimal vitamin D levels. Why is Muhammad Ali the greatest? No doubt his skill and showmanship played the largest part, but so I bet did his heavy bones. The tragedy was that he went on to suffer an illness thought to be related to vitamin D deficiency; Parkinson's disease.

A 1989 letter to the sports editor of *The New York Times* from a black African man made an interesting point that there should be no politically correct fear in embracing the fact that blacks are often top athletes.[127] One of his other personal observations was that Africans excel academically more frequently than African-Americans. If true, why is this? Black people living where they are designed to be not only enjoy better diets consisting of much less processed food when not in poverty, they also enjoy more sunlight despite the hindrance of clothes and indoor living. I would not be surprised if the infrequent participation of South Asians in sports with any degree of aggression is because of having the worst vitamin D levels despite similar production ease to whites. Bangladesh, India and Pakistan are typically cricketing nations. There are no top drawer Asian footballers in the UK, or even heavyweight boxers who need to attain weight through a balance of bone and muscle mass.

So what am I saying? That immigrants who arrived via high-speed transport, and their descendants, should go 'home' for their own benefit? No. Politics, economics and desire are all valid reasons to move around. What I am implying is, if you were designed for a cold climate and you live in the opposite, you should enjoy the sun regularly but make sure not to burn. If you were designed for a warmer climate but were put under grey clouds, you should be taking vitamin D. As most people cannot get reasonable UVB exposure these days the only way to ensure mental and physical equality would be for us to all share an optimal level of vitamin D through supplementation and food fortification. Affirmative action policies in the workplace could rightly be dismantled as it is better to have equal competition rather than forced quota filling.

You may have seen a picture portraying human evolution

when you were at school. It shows the development of monkey into mankind, marked by increased height and better posture. If we do not address the vitamin D deficiency pandemic the next figure to be drawn into such pictures will be that of a very small man with a curved spine, possibly lying with eyes closed on the floor.

6. Cholesterol & Heart Disease

The lipid hypothesis is the theory that too much cholesterol – a lipid – in the blood can narrow the arteries and produce heart disease.[128] The hypothesis arose in the early twentieth century, gained traction in the middle of it and is now seen as an irrefutable fact.[129]

It was conceived when it was noted that rabbits fed cholesterol developed thickened arteries. The first problem with this is that lab animals are confined for months and are not provided any source of UVB from which they could produce vitamin D via fur or skin cholesterol. Secondly, the amount of cholesterol given to these animals was too excessive. A paper thirteen years later in 1926, however, found normal cholesterol readings in some rabbits with arterial disease. More interesting was that high cholesterol and arterial disease appeared together when rabbits were fed a diet with excessive protein.[130] Perhaps the cholesterol elevation was a response to deal with the probable inflammation caused by a high-protein diet, coupled with the evident stress of being a lab animal.

Today the standard treatment for preventing heart disease remains the restriction of saturated fat and cholesterol-containing foods, and getting enough exercise. If these measures aren't enough, cholesterol-lowering drugs called statins are prescribed. The effectiveness of these drugs[131] has led to criticism of the hypothesis meeting ridicule.

So popular is the theory that you can find cholesterol-lowering foods in supermarkets, often based on plant stanols. There had even been a suggestion to put statins in British drinking water due to their apparent safety.[132] But not everyone prescribed the drugs has praised them as they have caused many debilitating side effects more commonly than thought, potentially outweighing their benefits. This is evidenced by media coverage of exceptional cases such as when people have experienced muscle wastage or memory loss. Our brains utilise a lot of cholesterol, so anything interfering with its production can lead to impaired brain function.[133]

It is important to note that cholesterol does have benefits and the mainstream view agrees that you need some of it. For a start, if you did not have any you would be unable to make vitamin D. It would be logical to assume, then, that there exists a recommended range for cholesterol values to let you know if your levels are *too low* (hypocholesterolaemia) as well as too high (hypercholesterolaemia). It appears not; not universally anyway.

I was twenty-seven when I had my cholesterol tested for the first time on a general blood check. I was slightly nervous of it because on my maternal side there is a strong history of heart disease. My grandfather died of a heart attack in his early fifties and my mother experienced heart failure at the same age. Furthermore, my father takes a statin. When my results arrived I was slightly dismayed that my cholesterol profile indeed showed me to be 'mildly' at risk. I assumed this risk would certainly increase as I aged. My GP did not prescribe a statin but handed me a British Heart Foundation leaflet to study, and advised that I *may* need to take a pill if diet change and exercise failed to reduce my level. It wasn't as helpful a read as I expected as there was little I could do to change my diet, neither do I drink or smoke. I consume very little processed foods, and though I am a regular meat eater, it is in small amounts, commonly with the fat removed. Additionally, I power walk with my brother for an hour per day and indulge in fast, aggressive drumming once per week for up to six hours. I have a body that I class as non-athletic slim muscular.

My serum (total) cholesterol level was 5.62 mmol/L (millimoles per litre), which is around the UK average according to one popular patient resource.[134] The US measures cholesterol in milligrams per decilitre which is achieved by multiplying mmol/L by 38.67, so in this case it's 217 mg/dL. For the rest of this chapter, though, I am going to stick to mmol/L, but as I'm focussing on general decreases or increases this shouldn't alienate some readers.

The following table is my morning fast result broken down – please note that the cholesterol guidelines set on my GP's computer were slightly generous compared to the then recommended national figures:

Table 6.1. My cholesterol profile, August 2007.

	Local UK GP guideline (mmol/L)	My result
Serum cholesterol	0.00-5.00	5.62 (High)
Non-HDL cholesterol	0.00-4.00	4.51 (High)
Serum HDL cholesterol	1.00>	1.11 (Normal)
Serum triglycerides	<1.7 (For fasting)	2.03 (High)
Serum cholesterol/HDL ratio	0.00-5.00	5.06 (High)

As you can see, three of the measurement guidelines start

from 0.00 – including total. While zero would be unachievable in living persons anyway, it is strange that if some cholesterol is good for us that the total is apparently allowed to be zero by any surgeries or hospitals. Similarly, there must be a point that "good" HDL cholesterol shouldn't exceed. Evidence of this is the shelved drug torcetrapib which reduced "bad" LDL as typical statins do but also raised HDL. The question is whether the failure of torcetrapib was down to unique side effects or the idea of artificially raising HDL itself.

HDL (high-density lipoprotein) is thought of as good cholesterol because it is believed to carry away non-good cholesterol from the arteries for disposal or reuse. An analogy could be that HDL are cholesterol binmen. If you don't have enough of them rubbish can accumulate in some areas, but if you have too many, those who feel redundant may enter your house and bin your valuables. LDL (low-density lipoprotein) and triglycerides are the villains because they are believed to clog arteries. The ILLUMINATE study, which aimed to assess the effectiveness of torcetrapib, pitted that drug plus atorvastatin against atorvastatin alone. In my opinion, pairing a drug which inhibits cholesterol production with one that promotes disposal is as bad an idea as giving laxatives to someone who is starving themselves. Torcetrapib was shelved because of too many deaths in the group who took both.[135] The desire to produce a good-cholesterol-raising drug came about to fill a hole in current treatment. While statins such as atorvastatin – commonly known as Lipitor, a best-selling drug[16] – have proved effective, they have not eradicated the spectre of heart disease which is why hopes have been pinned on the raising of HDL alongside.

A curious observation in the prescription of statins is that they are also advised for those with low or "normal" LDL and serum cholesterol levels *plus* extra risk factors, such as family history or lifestyle, and, particularly, above average levels of CRP (C-reactive protein) which indicates inflammation. It seems that in these people that statins are still effective.[136] It appears clear, then, that a drug which is effective in people with low or high cholesterol and affects inflammation works not because it reduces cholesterol.

In 2006 Dr. David Grimes published in *The Lancet* the question 'Are statins analogues of vitamin D?'[137] An analogue in this case is a virtual clone. A year after this – when I had my cholesterol tested – I myself wondered if there was a link between cholesterol and vitamin D, as aside from my borderline high cholesterol profile I found out I was also vitamin D deficient; just months after my brother had been put on the substance to treat his osteomalacia. These were the only two evident problems in my general blood test results at the time. I was unaware of Grimes's paper for a long period and egotistically believed that I had come up with the hypothesis first. I, however, had doubts about my simple conclusion until the discovery that it had already formed in a much-learned mind; I had worried that I misread the link between cholesterol in the skin and vitamin D.

A paper which raised my eyebrows further stated that atorvastatin increases vitamin D levels.[17] However, the study sponsored by the manufacturers of Lipitor, Pfizer, noted that "this increase could explain *some* [emphasis added] of the beneficial effects of atorvastatin at the cardiovascular level that are unrelated to cholesterol levels." Another study found that taking vitamin D alongside atorvastatin resulted in lower levels of the latter in the blood, yet LDL and serum cholesterol reduction were still apparent.[138] Therefore, it seems that the core beneficial effect of atorvastatin is increased vitamin D levels and taking both leads to the 'real deal' being victor in the body. Activated vitamin D – known as 1,25D – is also anti-inflammatory[139] which would make it ideal for lowering CRP.

It would seem in this case that cholesterol is inhibited because the liver, perhaps through the brain, realises it does not have to create as much to be sent to the skin for conversion as vitamin D has entered orally. As I will detail shortly, I found effective supplementation increased my HDL level. It may have risen simply because my body could actually afford to dispose of some "bad" cholesterol by its own accord.

Not all statins increase vitamin D levels though, an example being Zocor (simvastatin).[140] But none of them would need to if they ape vitamin D through another – non-analogue – method. Studies are continuing to be done on statins because not all of their mechanisms are clear. Pfizer cannot claim to know how Lipitor entirely works.

If statins are indeed solely vitamin D alternatives, then what better than to take the free or cheap original with little or no side effects? Backing this up is a study which found that statins help prevent strokes[141] despite cholesterol having no evident association with the condition. Also, as mentioned in the *Skeletal Effects* chapter, statins seem to curiously benefit bones. Their use prior to acquiring a serious head injury even appears to result in better survival and recovery than if not on a statin.[142] Can they prevent prostate cancer? Likely.[143] This is a master of many trades. One non-synthetic statin called Mevacor (lovastatin) is even derived from oyster mushrooms which can contain high levels of vitamin D – albeit as D2 which is natural to fungus.[144]

Men who are deficient in testosterone have a higher prevalence of heart disease.[145] What's interesting is that vitamin D appears to boost testosterone,[33] and effective testosterone therapy itself seems to positively modify cholesterol profiles and protects against heart disease.[146] This suggests that, at least in men, some of the benefits of vitamin D or sunlight itself such as improved insulin resistance, better bone density and muscle strength are brought on through raising testosterone. Worryingly, statins appear to reduce testosterone[147] which may explain some of their negative side effects. Note that testosterone is also produced from cholesterol.

In women, oestrogen – which too is made from cholesterol – reduces LDL and raises HDL.[148] However, this is not an endorsement of HRT (hormone replacement therapy) for post-menopausal women as they could be better off sticking with natural vitamin D orally or through skin conversion to protect their bodies from various problems such as osteoporosis, heart disease and cancer.

What throws a larger spanner at the lipid hypothesis is a finding by Dr. Malcolm Kendrick, author of *The Great Cholesterol Con* (John Blake Publishing 2008). On YouTube.com Kendrick narrates over a line graph that compares average male total cholesterol levels with heart disease death rates in most European countries, alongside that of Australian Aborigines. The data is from the World Health Organisation's MONICA (MONItoring trends and determinants in CArdiovascular disease) study.[149] What Kendrick highlighted was that there is no correlation between cholesterol levels and heart disease. What is of interest, though, is that Australian Aborigines have the highest rate of heart disease in the world and the least cholesterol, while the Swiss have virtually the opposite.

What this shows is that low cholesterol is not necessarily advantageous. We know that vitamin D deficiency is pandemic so it is very unlikely that the Aborigines' cholesterol levels are low because of significant vitamin D in their bodies, plus very few live as they did prior to European colonisation. High cholesterol in the Swiss could be seen as perfectly normal if it co-exists with sufficient or optimal vitamin D levels; at the very least it presents ample opportunity to make vitamin D. What should assure them is that low HDL and low serum cholesterol are frequently observed in critically ill infected people.[150]

Vitamin D deficiency doesn't necessarily indicate inflammation, but an inability to deal with it. This is probably why Kendrick's graph shows no pattern. France and Poland present similar levels of cholesterol but the former experience less heart disease. It could be that dietary factors other than saturated fats and cholesterol play a part in invoking inflammation, or that there are things in the French diet which compensate for vitamin D deficiency; or that they have more HDL. The direct cause of inflammation, though, is not something I feel able to deduce, but the fact that the French stereotypically value better quality food, as opposed to the processed food popular in England and America, may indicate where investigation should be directed. Unnatural products could even be detrimental to a vitamin D-replete body. Cholesterol sceptics like Kendrick aren't obliged to offer an explanation as to the causes of heart disease but he favours avoiding drug and alcohol misuse, reducing stress and taking regular exercise. Men were investigated by him as we are the current main consumers of statins.

We should be careful, however, of painting produce like wine as beneficial in small amounts. Alcoholism is always a theoretical risk to whoever drink is introduced.

Furthermore, despite some investigation, there is no known mechanism for how a little alcohol could be heart-protective. A 1997 study from America that seems to support moderate drinking also reported that blacks still suffer as much heart disease with two drinks per day. Former drinkers also present more heart disease[151] and we could say that such people may have become less outgoing and/or quit because of damage acquired. In the UK the majority of teetotallers would undoubtedly be Muslim, so it's a pure guess to believe that their abstinence is what places them at higher risk of heart disease over other factors. If anything, even one drink daily is perhaps more deleterious to people with severe vitamin D deficiency.

Another ace card that can be played is the paradox that cocaine addicts report low cholesterol levels[152] but are highly likely to suffer heart disease.[153] The key issue in regards to the lipid hypothesis, then, is that cholesterol levels seem largely irrelevant when the body is stocked with an anti-inflammatory.

So, what is clogging arteries then? You may have seen pictures of a yellow substance lining the walls of a tube-like artery, but this is not necessarily cholesterol. Few of you will have heard of arterial calcification which is when calcium obstructs arteries. There are two interdependent reasons as to why this would happen. Firstly, if vitamin D and calcium intake are low, parathyroid hormone will release calcium from the bones to satisfy the blood level. Secondly, a lack of vitamin K will not help to drive the excess away from arteries – and the excess may even come from heavy calcium supplementation. Calcification as a cause of heart disease may be distinct from inflammatory causes or accompany it. Osteoporosis is a frequent companion of the illness for reasons you can fathom, and a small study found that taking a bone-strengthening drug with atorvastatin leads to a greater heart benefit,[154] presumably because the former allows the latter to concentrate on fighting inflammation with its limited vitamin D raising.

Like myself, many people are advised to modify their diet and lifestyle before being offered a statin. As far as I know this almost always proves unsuccessful given the popularity of Lipitor alone – now cheaper via off-patent competition. Even if you decrease consumption of cholesterol-containing foods your liver could simply make more of it to even the balance. Cholesterol production is not an illness and the amount produced in the vast majority of people is normal. It could be possible, however, that certain processed foods or bad bacteria trigger inflammation which leads to increased cholesterol production in hopes of conversion to extra vitamin D. In regards to exercise, it is worth investigating if those who do experience a change in cholesterol levels are undertaking more *outdoor* activity than previously. If it's proven that indoor physical activity doesn't reduce cholesterol as much, lounging in the sun could be effective alone. That is not to say that you shouldn't exercise.

Months after my mother suffered anaemia-triggered heart failure in late 2002 – and I would like to add that on hospital admission she was said to have very low cholesterol which later rose acceptably – she decided to visit Pakistan alone for the first time in over twenty years, worrying that she would not have another opportunity to do so. While still very weak at that point, the brief holiday did wonders. Though she remained fully clothed – but doesn't ever wear a burqa or hijab etc. – and mostly stayed within buildings, she would have got more incidental UVB exposure than is possible in England. Resultantly she reported feeling more energetic, though I cannot divorce the fact that respite from an autistic son also helped.

People diagnosed with FH (familial hypercholesterolaemia) are said to suffer from much higher cholesterol levels than most. The condition appears to be hereditary. As in most people, the elevation does not typically produce symptoms but some sufferers of FH present cholesterol deposits in the joints prior to the development of any heart problems.[155] In my view these deposits are not necessarily mostly composed of cholesterol but calcium, indicating a disordered bone metabolism that may be remedied by vitamins D and K. Asymptomatic FH sufferers may simply have a quirk where the liver produces more cholesterol than normal for no reason without it being harmful. Or they are invoking inflammation by some means.

When I had my cholesterol tested again in 2008 I expected to be told to return in the morning after a twelve-hour fast as previously, but was surprised that my blood was taken there and then. This was at a hospital rather than with my GP. I since learned that it might not be necessary to fast for cholesterol tests and that triglycerides appear to have no predictive value.[156] The hospital may have known this before it was announced in the press. I didn't observe a dramatic change after a year on 5000 IU of vitamin D3, but I was not disappointed as my cholesterol profile had 'improved', even though my dose had only just pushed me into the beginning of sufficiency. The table below shows the amount of difference from the previous year's test. Note that higher HDL is a good thing.

Table 6.2. My cholesterol profile, September 2008 vs. August 2007.

	Result (mmol/L)	Change
Serum cholesterol	5.30 (High)	-0.32
Non-HDL cholesterol	3.30 (Normal)	-1.21
Serum HDL cholesterol	1.20 (Normal)	+0.09
Serum triglycerides	1.70 (High)	-0.33
Serum cholesterol/HDL ratio	4.40 (Normal)	-0.66

On second glance, however, I noticed something odd. My GP's computer calculates serum cholesterol as a simple addition of HDL with LDL – confirmed by the following year's result – whereas my hospital factors in triglycerides. Technically, the GP should be correct if triglycerides can be disregarded, but I would imagine that the hospital's formula is the norm. Supposing my GP is correct, my serum cholesterol here should have been 4.50 mmol/L, which is a bigger reduction. If wrong, my original serum cholesterol must have been around 7 mmol/L. Regardless, I will respect the hospital's calculations where it appears here – and their slight differences in recommended ranges – even though it obfuscates matters; to emphasise the farce. But if I were to exclude triglycerides from all of the hospital results in this chapter, small rises and falls away from the 2007 total would still be apparent.

Over the following twelve months I doubled my dose by taking one 50,000 IU capsule every five days. Then my cholesterol was measured again – fasted – by my GP, and it was amazingly different to two years prior. My GP did not print a prescription nor give a lecture. Neither did she question how I pulled off such a feat. My serum cholesterol was now way below UK average, if such a thing really matters. In the table below I have compared this profile with my initial one.

Table 6.3. My cholesterol profile, September 2009 vs. August 2007.

	Result (mmol/L)	Change
Serum cholesterol	4.95 (Normal)	-0.67
Non-HDL cholesterol	3.68 (Normal)	-0.83
Serum HDL cholesterol	1.27 (Normal)	+0.16
Serum triglycerides	1.34 (Normal)	-0.69
Serum cholesterol/HDL ratio	3.90 (Normal)	-1.16

Only one part of my cholesterol profile was insignificantly high and that was a measurement *only* taken on my 2009 test. This was serum LDL cholesterol at 3.07 mmol/L (ideal range: 0.00-3.00). I'm slightly confused by this as the label suggests that it is the same thing as non-HDL cholesterol, but I'll discount it anyway for the other higher figure of 3.68 which was a slight increase from 2008. This is my reason for not labelling non-HDL as LDL in these tables. My vitamin D level this time, however, had finally entered optimal range in accordance with cutting-edge US guidelines.

Regardless, I still have a dispute with what constitutes as normal cholesterol levels. For example, high serum cholesterol or ratio likely means nothing as long as they comprise of many *positive* large LDL particles over fewer negative small ones.[157] Therefore, quality not quantity is the real issue. It is unfortunate that LDL particle size is not commonly measured. I can only assume that my particle size had improved from before as a study shows that as triglycerides lower LDL particle size increases.[158] Small particles are associated with greater risk of heart disease. That said, if the usefulness of triglycerides is in doubt I can't be certain I have large LDL particles.

It was upon this result that I became really convinced that vitamin D affects cholesterol measurements while diet and exercise probably only bring benefit if, for example, frequent dining of fish and the donning of a t-shirt and shorts outside are involved. Stock pre-statin advice would also partly bemuse vegetarians or vegans who can't make any 'realistic' dietary changes.

Throughout 2010 I dropped down 3000 units to 7000 IU to see if my cholesterol profile would look less favourable. I also started taking 5000 mcg of vitamin B12, in preferred methylcobalamin form, once every four days to correct a diagnosed low level while seemingly being asymptomatic. 90 mcg daily of vitamin K2 was another addition, as stated in *Skeletal Effects*. This time my prediction didn't get a chance to breathe: my vitamin D level had *increased* by 6 nmol/L (2.4 ng/mL); plus, aside from raised triglycerides, there appeared no big change in my cholesterol profile – although it was towards the negative, which was unavoidable given that my hospital factors triglycerides into serum cholesterol.

Table 6.4. My cholesterol profile, September 2010 vs. September 2009.

	Result (mmol/L)	Change
Serum cholesterol	6.10 (High)	+1.15
Non-HDL cholesterol	3.50 (Normal)	-0.18
Serum HDL cholesterol	1.20 (Normal)	-0.07
Serum triglycerides	3.10 (High)	+1.76
Serum cholesterol/HDL ratio	5.10 (High)	+1.20

What this shows is that I no longer need too high a dose to sustain my vitamin D level. This highlights why annual vitamin D testing at minimum is important as your requirements may change. My body seems to no longer use up reserves immediately, which is a good sign. If triglycerides, as previously discussed, don't have much impact on cardiovascular risk, the high value here erroneously inflated my serum cholesterol and ratio. The volatility of triglycerides – e.g. in regards to food – might vindicate ignorance of them. Certainly, however, triglycerides could predict something if they remain constantly high or low. HDL and LDL seem to be affected virtually predictably by vitamin D, and raising of the former will raise serum cholesterol and ratio while being a positive contribution.[159]

One other curious observation is that my vitamin D level this time was said to be "perfect" by a different hospital consultant, despite being a bit higher than in the previous year in which I was told to halve my vitamin D intake. Having not been given a reference range at this time I'm not sure if the upper end of acceptable had been raised, at least by the London hospital in question.

In my final year of observation, in which the only supplements I took were B12 and D3, – the result of the latter somewhat worrying my doctor whom I lied to about my 'large' dose – my fasted results were as follows; perhaps ignore the triglycerides and note the HDL level:

Table 6.5. My cholesterol profile, October 2011 vs. September 2009.

	Result (mmol/L)	Change
Serum cholesterol	6.30 (High)	+1.35
Non-HDL cholesterol	4.00 (High, by hospital reference)	+0.32
Serum HDL cholesterol	1.30 (Normal)	+0.03
Serum triglycerides	2.20 (High, by GP reference)	+0.86
Serum cholesterol/HDL ratio	4.80 (Normal)	+0.90

The hospital recommended a GP consultation about my serum cholesterol level but only half-heartedly. Following this test – and ignoring the recommendation – I reduced my dosage to 4000 IU daily, which I believe is all I need to keep my vitamin D level around 150 nmol/L (60 ng/mL). Of course, this isn't set in stone if it appears I need more or less in future. In any case, I have demonstrated that 12,500 IU daily doesn't necessarily push an optimal person into toxicity within a season, so a gravely deficient person should not at all fear this dose as it could just quickly winch them into optimality.

I have convinced myself to never consider statins. Five years worth of personal observation is enough for me. But you would need to measure what happens in your own body as I cannot guarantee that you will share my experience. I could have provided better evidence of my blood results but generic-looking printouts should not convince you – only your own trial and observation should; and this is a safe experiment to do as long as you monitor your vitamin D level. If you need further goading, consider that a randomised double-blind clinical trial in 2011 showed that a vitamin D-fortified yoghurt drink raises HDL and reduces LDL and serum cholesterol in diabetics.[160]

Other than HDL, none of my cholesterol measurements show a constant enough trend to warrant a graph. Unpredictable triglycerides appear to have soiled my serum cholesterol and ratio levels, as has lack of consensus between my GP and hospital. On average, though, my LDL did drop modestly over the years, and the one year where my HDL dropped seems to be due to lower intake, despite a slightly higher vitamin D level than in the year prior.

Graph 6.1.

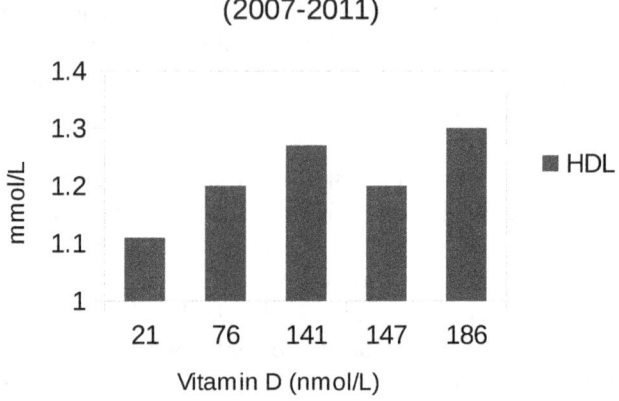

My vitamin D and HDL levels over 5 years

(2007-2011)

I must point out that, apart from taking vitamin D and additional supplements, over the years I did not undertake more exercise than previously or modify my diet. It is still possible that my cholesterol changes were a fluke but I find it convincing that my profile largely changed positively as my vitamin D intake rose. As stated a little further back, do not let increased serum cholesterol or ratio dishearten you as their major contributor could be desirable HDL as well as highly variable triglycerides.

It would be reasonable to wonder if I would consider one or two more follow-up observations where I allow myself to become deficient again, but, believing what I believe, I do not want to risk inviting illness even for a short period. I would much rather chance toxicity once more. Maybe you are braver?

Another thorn to disclose is that when my brother had his vitamin D and cholesterol checked twice – fasted – within a year by our GP, his profile was negatively impacted at a higher vitamin D level; HDL had decreased a few points while everything else rose. Why this is, I do not know, but the finding that the absence of certain gut bacteria may affect statin efficacy[161] could ring a bell with him; that is to say, would statins even help him considering that he had a bowel problem which still requires medicinal maintenance? I had also given him high-strength fish oil capsules as his initial cholesterol profile was less favourable than my first one. Abandoning vitamin D in his case, though, is out of the question as it is too crucial to his well-being in other areas.

Also, I should've been expected to have extremely high, LDL-laden serum cholesterol when severely vitamin D deficient.

It is not suggested that people on statins throw them away and suddenly take vitamin D only since more studies are needed. However, if like me you are offered a chance at redemption following a cholesterol test, it is worth checking your vitamin D level and perhaps addressing it before your next blood tests. If you also have the ability to get your LDL particle size checked, do so. If your cholesterol levels are entirely "normal" you should figure out why this is and pass the advice on to others. Are your levels better in the summer?

If you're still scared of taking vitamin D it might be worthwhile eating ketchup or drinking tomato juice as they appear to at least cut LDL[162] which would satisfy any doctor obsessed with that alone. It would also cost less and perhaps be safer than pills from the pharmacy.

The 9 August 2003 edition of *New Scientist* magazine ('Why Sunshine Is Good For You') referred to cholesterol in the skin as a "precursor chemical" that becomes vitamin D upon exposure to sunlight, and even now it's not often revealed to the public what the chemical in question is. If it were, conceivably more people would share my epiphany.

I've not covered hypertension (sustained high blood pressure) here but I believe that standard random measuring provides little value. Blood pressure varies throughout the day for a number of reasons such as anxiety or excitement, so only 48-hour monitoring with a reliable portable device in a relaxed home environment could identify true hypertension. Regardless, there is a suggestion that vitamin D helps to keep blood pressure lower on average,[163] perhaps partly because blood doesn't need to fight in pumping through calcium-free arteries; and a study shows that black people are more likely to suffer from hypertension than whites, feasibly due to a vitamin D disparity.[164]

To summarise, it's perhaps not cholesterol reduction that you should be worried about, rather making sure that it's converted or inhibited by its own accord. At the end of the day, inflammation and arterial calcification seem to be the true villains of heart disease.

Interview: Dr. David Grimes

Dr. David Grimes is a consultant physician specialising in gastroenterology in Blackburn hospitals. He holds an MD from The University of Manchester and is the author of Vitamin D and Cholesterol: The importance of the sun. *His review 'Are statins analogues of vitamin D?' featured in* The Lancet.

What made you doubt the cholesterol hypothesis of heart disease?
I suppose it was personal observation, the fact that the hypothesis simply didn't fit in with what I was seeing; many people with heart disease have normal cholesterol. I read into it in great detail and it simply doesn't make sense. Statins act in ways other than on cholesterol.

You believe that statins are probably effective because they raise vitamin D levels, but could they work by some other mechanism?
The mechanism they work by has something to do with vitamin D. They either activate vitamin D receptors or vitamin D responsive elements in the genome, but whatever they do has some link with vitamin D. I'm quite sure of that.

If high cholesterol is not the cause of coronary heart disease, what do you think is?
A bacterial or viral infection. Probably Chlamydophila pneumoniae which is a non-free-living bacterium.

If bacteria can cause heart disease, is it plausible that the link with dental health might be unnoticeable pieces of decaying food stuck in the teeth for a long time?

No. It's likely through respiratory tract infection. That seems to kick off coronary heart disease. There's a possibility it comes through the teeth but I think the main thing is the respiratory tract.

To your knowledge, how mild and rare are statin side effects?

There's surprisingly few. Sometimes they're intolerable, but not dangerous. They're reversible.

What do your colleagues make of your resistance to conventional thinking?

Many are sympathetic but the vast majority don't have an opinion because they've not read into it. Scepticism based on ignorance is not very good, and the ignorance is astounding. People just accept what they're told and don't question it.

The vested interests are immense. The amount of money in statins is immense. And, of course, they fund not just the companies and shareholders but also medical education. Furthermore, a lot of research departments depend on statin and cholesterol income.

Have you noticed a difference over the years in the age and severity of people affected with heart disease?

Coronary heart disease is a 20th century epidemic and it's almost gone. It doesn't occur, effectively, in young people, it tends now to occur only in the old; it's a cohort effect. As older people become older and die off the disease will disappear. It's amazing. It's nothing like as bad as it used to be.

When I was a young doctor we used to see a lot of middle-aged men, even young men, with severe coronary heart disease, and now we just see a mild disease in old people. It's a big change. People will say that's because of modern preventive medicine but that's nonsense.

Do you think it's possible for humans to evolve to not need vitamin D or very much of it?
You can't evolve, you've got to have a mutation. What scientists could do is a bit of genetic engineering from mice, utilising the mouse gene that has a different pathway.

Would full-body tattoos and burn scars impede vitamin D synthesis?
Tattoos will. I've never thought about burn scars but I would imagine so, though people aren't likely to expose them anyway. Lots of tattoos are also not kept on show.

Is fish oil a necessary thing to take with vitamin D in order for good heart health?
I think it all depends on how much sun you get. If you don't get much sun you need a lot of fish oil. But people who get plenty of sun, that's all they need. [*I'm not sure if Dr. Grimes differentiated between fish oil and vitamin D-containing cod liver oil.*]

Is over-nutrition an exclusive cause of obesity, if not, what do you think other causes are, and does that impact heart disease development?
Difficult to know. Over-nutrition is interesting. I got the figures out and looked at diet during the past sixty years in the UK and found food intake has gone down overall. The story of obesity is greatly exaggerated but I think a lot of it is lack of physical exercise. I think that is the

major factor actually, in childhood particularly.

Astronauts can lose some height during space missions, is this partly due to no opportunity to make vitamin D and ineffective supplementation?

It's probably osteoporosis due to bone disuse which is not vitamin D-related. [This?] osteoporosis has got nothing to do with vitamin D.

Do your patients often present multiple instances of vitamin D deficiency-related illness, or is it usually one thing?

It can be the one illness of bone disease but usually it's a combination of illnesses like heart disease, diabetes, liver disease and Crohn's disease.

Tuberculosis is an AIDS-defining illness and a vitamin D deficiency illness. Do you think there's any link between both backdrops?

There are two causes of acquired immunodeficiency syndrome: one of them is HIV and the other is vitamin D deficiency.

Susceptibility to disease can be inherited, but are we placing less importance on environment?

Well, yes. Infection runs in families, for example, tuberculosis and syphilis would run in families through close living contact. Hepatitis B virus can be passed from mother to baby during the process of birth by mixing of the blood, as noted in China.

Believe it or not, about 50% of our genome is from viruses, and nobody knows how long they've been there and what they're doing there. Viruses have a big effect and they could be a part of solutions as well as problems.

For information on his book visit vitamin-d-deficiency.co.uk

7. HIV/AIDS

Vitamin D deficiency is common in HIV-(human immunodeficiency virus)-positive patients,[165] however, it is as yet uncertain if the problem is more marked in this group compared to the general worldwide population; only a small study so far has found that the HIV+ have lower levels than the HIV-.[166] Low vitamin D, though, does appear to accelerate the development of AIDS (acquired immune deficiency syndrome).[167]

I must state up front that after researching the links exhaustively I have come to classify myself as an AIDS Rethinker. This means I dispute the orthodox belief that a retrovirus – a virus which relies on a host cell for infection – called HIV is the cause of AIDS. A more popular term used to describe AIDS Rethinkers is denialists. This is employed in an effort to draw misguided comparisons with Holocaust deniers. The branding has been effective in making Rethinkers seem as if they are composed of negligent and murderous individuals when nothing could be further from the truth. I do not believe that there is a conspiracy, just that, as with the cholesterol hypothesis, there are good reasons to doubt the accepted wisdom.

I acknowledge that the views expressed here could make some readers feel I have crossed a line, which is why I present them with the caveat that even if you disagree with what I've written, it remains plausible that vitamin D could help to treat HIV/AIDS under a mainstream understanding.

As far as I know, I am virtually alone in having

married vitamin D reassessment with AIDS Rethinking. At best, this chapter should be used to stimulate debate rather than be directly acted upon.

The story of AIDS began in the early 1980s when a cluster of gay American men developed either a cancer called Kaposi's sarcoma or PCP (Pneumocystis pneumonia). It was believed that a hedonistic attitude to their sexuality – which may have included the use of recreational drugs called alkyl nitrates ("poppers") – was to blame,[168] and this led to the coining of an early acronym called GRID (gay-related immune deficiency).[169] However, when other groups of people began presenting the same diseases[170] the acronym had to be revised. AIDS was the one that stuck and the hunt was on for an infectious cause.

In 1984 it seemed that hunt was over when the American secretary for health announced via press conference that scientist Robert Gallo had found the "probable cause" of AIDS, a variant of a human cancer virus called HTLV-III (human T-lymphotropic virus type III).[171] HTLV-III was not discovered by Gallo – that accolade goes to a group of French scientists led by Luc Montagnier[172] who called the virus LAV (lymphadenopathy-associated virus) a year earlier – but it was Gallo who appeared to demonstrate that the virus, renamed HIV, could be the cause of AIDS. There was initial controversy as to why the Gallo-found virus looked too identical to Montagnier's, but this was explained by a sample from Montagnier's lab having contaminated what Gallo was working on.[173] Following years of wrangles over credit both men reached a truce and are now equally regarded as pioneers of HIV/AIDS science.

With relief it was believed that a vaccine would be available within two years. Twenty-eight years later there is still no vaccine, only drugs alleged to maintain life. Gallo's work had not been scrutinised by fellow scientists before the press conference, but the razzmatazz relayed by rolling cameras and newsprint cemented the "probable cause" as definitive truth.

The reason why many believe the HIV/AIDS story is simple. Most of us are not affected by it and never will be, so few care to question. Many in the developed world do not even know where their nearest genitourinary clinic is to go for a test, and only the most persecuted groups will take the time to seek them out; possibly entering a self-fulfilling prophecy. British hospitals uncommonly have departments that deal specifically with HIV, – notably excluding London's Chelsea and Westminster Hospital which houses Europe's largest genitourinary/HIV clinic – nor are there poster campaigns in GP surgeries to regularly make people fear. Morbid television campaigns are also no longer repeated. All the majority feel is sympathy for those afflicted and trust that those in charge know what they're doing. But as with the lipid hypothesis you need to examine the data. Even reading mainstream HIV/AIDS literature alone with an open mind should make you doubtful.

The first problem with the HIV/AIDS hypothesis is the HIV test itself. Many people assume that it looks for the virus in the blood when in fact it looks for antibodies to it. The presence of antibodies can indirectly confirm that a particular virus *was* in the body, but not necessarily if it currently is,[174] or even if it is active. Similarly, antibodies to peanut proteins do not suggest you have peanuts in your gut or that you clinically react to them; like in myself. A way to visualise antibodies is as hitmen sent by the immune system to deal with specific threats. Their production is a function of adaptive immunity, which is plan B to general, innate, non-antibody immunity. If you test HIV+, your body could be keeping the virus in check or it has entirely neutralised it. Certainly, if a HIV vaccine were available it would make everyone HIV+ and necessitate tests that actually confirm the presence and activation of the virus – yet HIV diagnoses are made on antibody tests alone which have not been authorised for this use, and are shown to be unreliable as you can flip between positive, negative or indeterminate on repeated testing.[175] An argument exists that being HIV+ does not mean you have *potent* antibodies against the virus, but if this is true, then someone with HIV should likely have AIDS on immediate infection, as opposed to in a time frame of around a decade or more.[176]

It is true that many illnesses are confirmed by antibody tests alone for convenience purposes, but these are validated by gold standard (supreme quality) testing, undisputed prior viral isolation and demonstrable, unambiguous, causation. The latter two will be discussed shortly.

Kary Mullis's PCR (polymerase chain reaction) test is used to determine "viral load", which means to estimate how much virus is in the blood from a sample. A high viral load suggests mass replication is occurring, leading to or implying, in this case, "full-blown AIDS." The problem with PCR here is that it amplifies DNA to aid conclusion. This is like putting a magnifying glass on an ant and calling it a cockroach. If HIV is as destructive as it is said to be, it should not need such magnification in order to be detected in AIDS patients; just like other viruses. Furthermore, PCR is not immune from producing invalid results.[177] It is also important to note that Mullis, a Nobel Laureate in chemistry, does not support the HIV/AIDS hypothesis.[178]

Additional support for AIDS Rethinking, oddly, comes indirectly from Montagnier himself who believes that HIV alone may not be enough to induce AIDS.[179] If true, this may support my belief that HIV positivity does not necessarily indicate prior or current HIV infection, but immunodeficiency in the form of extreme vitamin D deficiency or insensitivity through hard drug use, malnutrition, malabsorption, or conversion issues. Such a physical state provides fertile ground for other threats to enter and for inflammation to develop.

An early treatment for HIV was the previously rejected cancer drug zidovudine (ZDV),[180] more commonly known as AZT (azidothymidine). Patient information for this drug reports one side effect to be immunodeficiency,[181] meaning it would be hard to know whether AIDS in an HIV patient is caused by HIV or AZT. This was a particular concern during the early years of the hypothesis when the drug was given at high doses before AIDS could ever develop. Today it is somewhat common practice to provide drug treatment simply when, if ever, a person starts showing signs of AIDS. This may be the core reason for less deaths on AZT now, alongside a decrease in dosage.[182]

Presently, AZT sometimes forms part of a drug cocktail called HAART (highly active antiretroviral therapy). Aside from the general toxicity of HAART, components of it, including AZT, have been found to reduce vitamin D levels while alternative treatment does not.[183] It is clear that reduction of an immunomodulator in immunodeficiency disease is not at all desirable. Regardless, if HAART were totally ineffective it would not be prescribed. One explanation of its efficacy is its antifungal properties,[184] which means that HAART should perhaps be changed to HAAFT to make clear that its few benefits have nothing to do with taming a retrovirus. Since cathelicidin works as a natural antifungal it stands to good reason that vitamin D, which helps to mass produce it,[185] would be part of a truly effective, gut-sparing and non-toxic therapy. Furthermore, as vitamin D has anti-tumour properties – revealed in *Popping Cancer* – it could deal with Kaposi's sarcoma.

It is true that people who test HIV+ on a chronic basis may be unwell or have a high potential to be, but contrary to a terrifying television campaign I witnessed as a child featuring a tombstone with nothing but 'AIDS' written on it, the predicted heterosexual epidemic in wealthy countries never materialised;[186] even though unprotected sex obviously never went out of fashion. In fact the key risk groups remain largely the same as ever, notably including the incarcerated.[187] This suggests that HIV is a prejudiced virus or that something else is common to these groups of people, whom I will outline. I suspect it is severe vitamin D deficiency and/or insensitivity which is easily argued as one cause of acquired immune deficiency syndrome, even if it may not qualify for the capitalised acronym. This is because vitamin D strengthens innate and adaptive immunity resulting in immune efficiency.

Another thing supporting the case that optimised immunomodulation is crucial to fighting HIV/AIDS is a mainstream-interpreted study which found that a lectin in bananas called BanLec could help in preventing HIV transmission.[188] BanLec is a potential immunomodulator.[189] This shows that nutrition can be key. But the amount of lectins needed and if it could outperform vitamin D is not currently known.

GcMAF is an experimental treatment also showing promise in treating a variety of immune-related problems, including HIV/AIDS. [gcmaf.eu] The MAF in its name shows that it is a 'macrophage activating factor'. Macrophages can be thought of as friendly monsters that chomp on invading threats and cellular debris. Interestingly, GcMAF has a telling alias: DBP-maf (the first three letters stand for vitamin D-binding protein; a vitamin D transporter not lacking in most people),[190] and one scientific thesis – which ponders whether HIV is actually part of the human genome, revealed through autoimmune antibody response to damaged cells, as opposed to being external and infectious – has this interesting thing to report: "Paricalcitol [a clone of active form vitamin D2] evoked a stimulatory response quite similar to that of GcMAF[,] and intracellular cAMP [cathelicidin, the body's own antibiotic] formation was strongest in the "FF/bb" genotype and non[-]significant in the homozygous "ff/BB" genotype."[191] The mention of genotypes refers to individual body responsiveness to vitamin D.

AIDS is seen as a major problem in sub-Saharan Africa thanks to media awareness. But a dubious observation is that endemic HIV infection in this region is due to a lack of education, leading to promiscuous, unprotected sex. Many have failed to notice that the area is largely Christian where the community mindset dictates to be faithful.

A rumour exists that HIV could have originated when Africans engaged in sexual practices with wild monkeys.[192] Not only is this tricky to believe, it reeks of racism. What is true about the region, though, is poverty leading to a lack of good nutrition and proper sanitation. Food deprivation itself will weaken a body, but it can also render vitamin D useless. If HIV is infectious it is strange how it neatly affects sub-Saharan Africa much more than its neighbours. The region is noted for its poor black population.

Nutritional deficiencies could also explain why gay men test HIV+ and fall ill. An unpublished theory by a HIV+ gay layman named Tony Lance – which expands on ideas by Vladimir Koliadin[193] – suggests that intestinal dysbiosis ("leaky gut syndrome") can result in ill health, partly because of an inability to absorb nutrients from food, leading to multiple deficiencies.[194] The cause of intestinal dysbiosis here is trauma to the gut from *excessive* and rough anal sex. Such behaviour is likely to be facilitated by recreational drug use, and, ironically, specific methods of anal cleansing to maintain hygiene for intercourse may also diminish gut function to some degree, perhaps through the destruction of gut VDR (vitamin D receptors). Spermicidal condoms (i.e. designed for vaginal intercourse) and lube might also play a detrimental role. Lance's theory certainly explains why many sufferers waste away in the same manner as starving people. If it is correct, then a method of repairing or at least improving gut function, – perhaps through stem cell therapy – alongside vitamin D repletion, could place affected gay men into the group known as long-term non-progressors; people who are HIV+ but develop AIDS at a much later date, if at all. The fact that a number of HIV+ people – frequently including females who engage in receptive anal sex[195] – remain free of AIDS, especially in absence of any mainstream treatments, could be due to how damaged the VDR is. It may be damaged enough to produce chronic HIV positivity, but not enough to ever produce AIDS; particularly if upon diagnosis a person then abstains from or limits further gut traumas.

Supporting this theory is a study on mice in whom it has been found that the VDR is a key player in regulating gut flora.[196] Though the results are meant to illuminate the cause of typical inflammatory bowel disorders, in my opinion they also shed light on AIDS. In the study the team looked at three groups of mice: ones with a functional VDR, ones that lacked it, and ones that were free from germs. Salmonella was introduced to all of them. Bear in mind that recurrent Salmonella infection is an AIDS-defining condition[197] before considering the following excerpt from a news piece on the study: "The scientists found that Salmonella was much more virulent and aggressive in mice in which the vitamin D receptor had been turned off. These mice showed higher levels of activity of inflammatory molecules, and they lost weight more quickly and were much more likely to die in response to infection."[198] That description of the VDR-disabled mice stereotypically portrays AIDS patients. Of course though, these are mice and not human beings, but the fact that they, like us, have intestines with vitamin D receptors shows that this is a good starting point to build upon. The additional fact of a defanged version of the Salmonella virus managing to produce *effective HIV antibodies* – seemingly – in mice who appear to have intact gut VDR[199] should be jaw-dropping evidence that the state of the gut is of immense importance. In Africa, Salmonella is endemic;[200] perhaps part fuelled by poor nutrition which can hinder the work of vitamin D.

I would like to add at this point that there is nothing to suggest that HIV knocks out the VDR.

Lance's paper also mentions glutathione deficiency, and we know from early in this book that vitamin D helps to produce glutathione[43] when nothing impedes it. Additionally, cytokines are repeatedly mentioned by Lance as having a positive influence when the gut is not compromised. When looking at a study concerning vitamin D and chronic heart failure, we see – even with the minuscule amount of vitamin D used – that the substance is able to promote anti-inflammatory cytokines and suppress pro-inflammatory ones.[201] Since virtually all organs have VDR we can reasonably assume that what's been observed in the heart can be observed in the gut.

To demonstrate that intestinal dysbiosis is a/the cause of AIDS via destruction of the gut VDR, research should be aimed at identifying and repairing any receptor anomaly, or providing substances that the VDR otherwise helps to produce. This would include friendly bacteria products – as suggested by Lance – in order to strike a balance with harmful bacteria in the gut to improve nutrient absorption. One study already confirms that probiotics have a favourable effect on the HIV+.[202] High-strength vitamin B12 supplementation or seasonal injections should also be considered to stave off AIDS-related dementia since diminished gut function makes B12 in food no longer enough.[203] Injections are effective as they bypass the gut, while 1% of an oral dose is absorbed through an alternative pathway, thus justifying a large intake.[204] Vitamin D deficiency in the first place may even account for B12 deficiency in the general population, perhaps due to an E.coli-triggered autoimmune attack on the specific stomach cells that absorb the nutrient.[205] Autoimmunity is explored in the *Influenza & Autoimmunity* chapter. Vitamin D itself would only be effective here if the VDR is not too damaged, though activated vitamin D may help with extremely careful dosing.

The crux, then, is that vitamin D *insensitivity* in the gut may lead to a HIV+ status as receptor dysfunction produces an inability to deal with the microbial proliferation that leads to inflammation and malnourishment. While vitamin D deficiency is a universal problem, most deficient people with a functional gut receptor likely have just enough activated vitamin D to fend off immense microbial overload. Some sufferers of inflammatory bowel disease, though, may get perilously close to temporal or chronic HIV positivity *because* of their gut condition.

Late singer and high-profile AIDS casualty Freddie Mercury seems to have – anecdotally – anally administered cocaine to avoid damaging his nose and throat, "However...the damage done to his intestinal lining was so severe that, in 1980, his rectum fell out... [And he] was finally forced to undergo expensive and painful surgery in 1982..."[206] Could it be that continued intestinal problems contributed to Mercury's death within a decade?

In order to curb the spread of HIV, drug abusers are advised that if they are to continue injecting recreational drugs they should not share needles. This lacklustre approach gives no real imperative to the drug user to quit as they believe they are safe with clean needles, but intravenous drug abuse itself is known to cause HIV positivity because they are immunosuppressive. A good example in the media is that of rock star Ozzy Osbourne who tested positive after having recently quit drugs, then negative on a later retest; presumably because the damage to his body – perhaps partly to his liver – was easily reversible. Interestingly, he was even told that his drug abuse may have been a contributory cause of the initial alarming result.[207] This begs the question of whether HIV is actually a virus at all as antibodies should stay with somebody for life, or at least a long duration to protect from immediate recurrent infection.

It should be noted too that hard recreational drugs such as cocaine can also cause gut perforation,[208] and this even affects the unborn children of female users.[209] This, then, could partly account for maternal HIV 'transmission'. Even without a direct physical impact on the gut, hard drug addiction stereotypically leads to an abandonment of adequate nutrition, which facilitates the development of general gut problems. It would be interesting to see, therefore, if anorexia nervosa sufferers frequently test positive; though ethical considerations would forbid such an experiment. Ethics, however, too, had forbidden all gay and bisexual men from donating blood despite the availability of screening.

A few years after Gallo's hypothesis entered public consciousness the first and still most prominent scientist to dispute that HIV causes AIDS was Peter Duesberg. He alleges that HIV is a harmless virus which piggybacks onto an already compromised immune system through the use of recreational and antiretroviral drugs or malnutrition.[210] Because of how large the propaganda machinery had become for the mainstream hypothesis, Duesberg found his funding slashed and associations with fellow scientists diminished. It is believed that his hypothesis is discredited,[211] but while there remains no effective treatment for HIV/AIDS it still shines like a beacon in the world of Rethinking.

Duesberg's hypothesis, however, is not the exclusive ideology of AIDS Rethinkers. The Perth Group led by Eleni Papadopulos believes that HIV has never even been properly isolated[212] and that testing positive could simply indicate hypergammaglobulinaemia, which means having too many antibodies to too many things; some of which might flag up as HIV in diagnostic test kits. This supports Lance's hypothesis since intestinal dysbiosis can allow many antigens – antibody-producing substances – into the bloodstream. General poor nutrition itself through lack of absorption or lack of food could also give rise to mass antibody production, and recent flu vaccination antibodies alone are a known cause of temporarily testing

HIV+.[213] Even worse, hard recreational drug use can lower cholesterol which in turn diminishes vitamin D production. This compromises first line innate immunity, leading the immune system to deal with the harmful effects of drugs and other antigens almost exclusively through antibody production.

The argument that HIV has never been isolated is bolstered by a statement from Montagnier himself that his group never purified the virus.[214] Purification is important because it separates the virus from other material. Retroviruses are known to 'band' at a certain area in a testing process but HIV purely has not been demonstrated there even by Gallo. Though there are electron microscope pictures of HIV, Papadopulos points out that they do not only show one thing; that HIV appears to be a mix of material.[215]

If you have ever seen pictures of HIV in print or on screen they will almost certainly have been computerised illustrations of what it alone is *alleged* to look like. What has rarely been pointed out is that these graphics appear in a range of different colours and barely similar designs. If you type 'HIV' into an image search engine you will find that electron microscope pictures are the least common amongst the results and – apart from repeat versions of the same image – none of the illustrations look alike. It has been stated that HIV mutates in order to avoid annihilation,[216] which would explain variation in the images; however, it is just as likely that there are many different material combinations which flag up as HIV.

Before the turn of the century in Ireland, the Lindsay Tribunal was set up to examine the extent of hepatitis C and HIV transmission in haemophiliacs and von Willebrand disease sufferers from blood products prior to

1985, when blood was not screened. While honourable, the subsequent report[217] would have you believe that only those with the mentioned bleeding disorders were given blood or one of its products when this was clearly not the case. An Irishwoman I know personally, who attended the tribunal, received a large blood transfusion in the early 1980s and recovered from a subsequent diagnosis of hepatitis C – but she did not catch HIV. I can find no documents that assess how many people, if any, without a bleeding disorder, – like herself – became HIV+ through Irish blood or one of its products. Interestingly, her treatment of synthetic interferon might've been better replaced with vitamin D which produces it naturally;[218] those who can rid hepatitis C without intervention could simply be vitamin D sufficient.

By nature, haemophiliacs continue to test HIV+ frequently despite screening of donated blood.[175] This begs the question of whether HIV was ever in the Irish blood supply; even if it were, the only thing that can be identified and removed are antibodies, which, theoretically, could work as a vaccine. Few question why HIV seems to selectively target haemophiliacs, almost exclusively through the use of dried blood products. HIV should not be able to survive long out of fluid.[219] Interestingly, drugs company Bayer was accused of knowingly selling such a product, contaminated with HIV, to haemophiliacs;[220] yet how this could happen has never been explained. Haemophiliacs simply tested HIV+ and a scapegoat was required. What strongly suggests vitamin D insensitivity, or perhaps lack of activation through reduced kidney function, is the fact that haemophiliacs commonly present low bone densities[221] and vitamin D has not proven effective for rickets in such sufferers.[222] Even the recommended daily allowance as ergocalciferol should show some effect.

Another powerful example is the plight of disabled children with HIV in Romanian orphanages. Media coverage unearthed abandonment, malnutrition, and the fact that the children rarely saw the light of day – yet dirty needles used to deliver nutritional supplements were blamed.[223] No evidence was provided to support this.

Much more devastating than the science itself is the unquestioning campaigns which enforce the prevailing view. Those who support the HIV/AIDS theory genuinely care about the people they wish to help, but their information is filtered by mainstream consensus. In the modern age more people listen to celebrities than politicians or scientists which is why they are often employed to raise awareness of particular campaigns. However, celebrity endorsement is often based on trust than careful examination of the science.

A case in point would be the controversial 2001 episode of the British satirical comedy *Brass Eye*. While the press picked up on the crass taste of a paedophilia special, the specific programme was not actually about paedophilia at all, rather, – ironically – over the top misinformed reactions from the media to certain issues. Its presenter Chris Morris did not glorify paedophilia but pointed out how irrational it was to think that paedophiles were present in large numbers in every area of England. Morris made an excellent mockery of local celebrities by tricking them enough to say things like "Genetically, paedophiles have more genes in common with crabs than they do with you and me. Now that is scientific fact. *There's no real evidence for it, but it is scientific fact.*"[224] While this is an extreme example where viewers easily understand that celebrities were being manipulated, who's to say that the likes of Bono, Bill Gates, Elton John and Annie Lennox, amongst others, haven't been unwittingly led astray? They certainly wouldn't have much time between campaigning and their day jobs to assess the science in depth, but even if they did, and they came to criticise it publicly, they would be ostracised in a similar fashion to other dissidents. It is a career faux pas. I'm not naming to shame here as these people do much else to help the deprived, but 'rich person's guilt' could lead one to think that only large amounts of money will help solve the seemingly unsolvable. They need to consider that African AIDS and poverty might just be one and the same.

Maintaining public sympathy is key to sustaining the hypothesis. It is little known that aside from wasting away some HIV patients can present obesity.[225] If the 1993 AIDS movie *Philadelphia* were to be remade and featured a protagonist who gained a lot of weight rather than lost it, it may not tug the heartstrings as much. The reason wasting seems less apparent now in the developed world is likely because of lower dosages of AZT, and at a later date.

Pregnant women are susceptible to 'falsely' testing HIV+[226] as their condition brings stress on the body. As discussed in the *Awakening* chapter, a vitamin D deficient mother may produce antibodies to her unborn child since half of the genetic material is unfamiliar to her overly cautious immune system. These antibodies may then cross-react as HIV. Children born to such women may also test HIV+ temporarily.

A study found that women who take vitamin D supplements are less likely to transmit HIV to their child.[227] What was not discussed was the possibility that such mothers are actually only *passing on* a strong immunomodulatory status. If a prenatal mother is vitamin D replete she may not produce antibodies to her offspring and, therefore, not pass them on. If she already has antibodies prior to or during pregnancy, these may still not be passed on if the foetus has no need for them. One reason babies can lose their HIV positivity in time could be because they inevitably consume milk products that may contain a small amount of vitamin D, which is enough for their systems. Children also soon enter the world of outdoor daylight where regular incidental exposure to a few uncovered areas can bring added benefit. Another thing in Lance's paper that supports this is the following quote: In *Mucosal Immun[ology]*, Cripps and Gleeson write: "The mucosal immune system is rapidly stimulated at birth by bacterial colonization of the mucosal and external surface...The initial bacterial colonization patterns in the gastrointestinal tract differ between breast and formula-fed infants; hence, so do the degree and nature of antigenic stimulation of the mucosal immune system." The book mentioned expresses the benefits of breast milk,[228] which, when coming from a vitamin D-sufficient mother, is undoubtedly preferable and in line with nature. Cow's milk is extremely low in vitamin D,[229] perhaps because dairy cows are often confined, and fortification policies differ worldwide. Plus, such large animals aren't adapted to many countries.

It has been ignored by the press that those who have unprotected vaginal intercourse with HIV+ people do not necessarily contract the status themselves. For example, even if high-profile AIDS Rethinker Christine Maggiore had HIV and passed it on to one of her children,[230] she clearly did not transmit it to her widowed husband who remains – in absence of any reportage or documents – HIV-free and in the best of health. To back this up, a study found that amongst over two hundred prostitutes, who are at high risk for contracting HIV, only female drug users tested positive. Very few non-drug-using transsexual males also tested positive,[231] perhaps as a result of intestinal dysbiosis. When we hear reports of male circumcision proving somewhat beneficial in preventing heterosexual HIV transmission, it is possible that the issue lay in foreskin hygiene; you may either snip it or you could make sure it's frequently cleaned to prevent the passing on of bacteria which may provoke antibodies that cross-react as HIV. If human males didn't cover their genitals most of the time I would imagine bacterial build-up would be less of a problem. Circumcision likely pre-dates Judaism and was perhaps seen as an easy solution to foreskin retraction problems and as a means of preventing any foreskin inflammation. Under the classic hypothesis, circumcision seems like nonsense because you have to acknowledge that semen still transmits HIV.

In late 2010 it was reported that German pop star Nadja Benaissa allegedly infected one of several sexual partners for which she was charged of negligence. Benaissa herself tested positive when she fell pregnant previously. Additionally, she is black and appears to be a former drug user.[232] Black people are more likely to test HIV+ than other racial groups,[233] and this fits neatly with vitamin D deficiency being a factor since darker skin coupled with clothing and indoor living makes them more susceptible. I do not know how many times Benaissa and her infected partner have been tested. A person is not usually retested once they are diagnosed HIV+.

An interesting *Chicago Tribune* article reported that a black, HIV+ former heroin user, once on the verge of death, lives a healthy life after sixteen years of being clean.[234] Was he retested? I doubt it; even if he were reconfirmed positive it might now be largely inconsequential in his case. The article also notes that HIV/AIDS patients have an increased risk of developing osteoporosis, which I believe is true for people who have an unaddressed immunity problem involving vitamin D. Is it surprising that Zimbabwean miners carry a significant burden of AIDS?[235] You can believe that they spend much of their time copulating or injecting, but I would place the blame on their working environment, amongst other variables.

While it is honourable to employ pesticides in malaria-hit regions like Africa and India, let it be known that some organochlorines may reduce vitamin D levels in humans.[236]

It is important to remember that no one dies from AIDS itself but opportunistic illnesses that flourish in a broken immune system. These comprise of at least eighteen previously known diseases.[237] If you contract one of them and are HIV- you are not said to be suffering from AIDS. Tuberculosis, which can be an AIDS-defining condition, is found in those lacking vitamin D,[238] those who take recreational drugs,[239] and the malnourished.[240] Homeless people in the developed world certainly could tick all three boxes.

When the HIV/AIDS hypothesis was crystallised only a handful of diseases were attributed as its outcome and consequent life expectancy was expected to be no more than a year. Given that the hypothesis had to be radically revised, this shows how desperate its existence is.

It is believed that HIV kills immune system 'soldiers' called T-cells but this has not been explicitly demonstrated.[241] Things get complicated when you hear it is possible to have AIDS via a decreased T-cell count without testing HIV+.[242] This could be blamed on unreliable tests for the virus or is proof that HIV is not an essential cause of AIDS. To play devil's advocate, if we were to say that HIV does exist, it is possible that HIV-free AIDS is not actually so, rather that the body couldn't produce HIV antibodies for some reason.

HIV/AIDS also fails a widely hailed test called Koch's postulates that determines if an infection is linked to a disease.[243] If HIV fulfilled the four postulates it would be found in *all* AIDS patients, be isolable and grow in pure culture, – which would give easy rise to an employable vaccine strain – cause disease in previously uninfected individuals, and be isolable again. For the latter two, HIV *sometimes* appears to cause AIDS and primary isolation is disputed, never mind secondary. Defenders of the hypothesis believe that Koch's postulates are outdated. In fairness, this may be true for some viral diseases but not those claimed as isolated.

One man is said to have been cured of HIV, which he had for a decade, when given a bone marrow transplant to treat leukaemia.[244] It is thought that this may have been a fluke even by doctors who treated the patient, but, if it wasn't, it could be interpreted that his HIV positivity was merely a non-specific prognosticator of the leukaemia, and that something in the transplant reactivated his disabled immunity which cleared the sign and manifestation. It is believed that a damaged version of a gene called CCR5 from the donor conferred a curative and protective effect from HIV. This version of CCR5 is found in a very small percentage of people largely consisting of Scandinavians,[245] who are fair-skinned and fish eaters. It is possible that a vitamin D-sufficient person's marrow was transplanted, and, additionally, the news of being free of HIV could have produced a positive psychological effect, leading to a sustained physiological one.

Statins for heart disease – which as stated in the

previous chapter could be clones of vitamin D – are shown to have anti-HIV activity too through control of intact CCR5;[246] making it behave like the damaged version. Controlled intact CCR5 could be more beneficial than its opposite.

In an observational study, people taking statins alongside HIV drugs had a 67% reduced risk of dying.[247] Perhaps if some were only taking statins that percentage could be much higher.

As with the cholesterol hypothesis, there is an obvious lack of desire from pharmaceutical companies to test if anything other than their products can treat the 'infected', the at risk, or the evidently suffering. This was confirmed by Montagnier himself in uncut footage concerning the sub-Saharan African epidemic from Brent Leung's multi-award winning – but little known – *House of Numbers* documentary.[248] That said, some claim Montagnier's poor grasp of English led to his being misunderstood.[249]

Perhaps the most compelling reason for investigation into alternative theories is the odd amount of resistance there is to those who challenge orthodox opinion. Decades before when science was less concerned with profiteering, criticism of any hypothesis was welcomed as it either helped strengthen a theory or made way for a better one. But now that AIDS has become a multi-billion-dollar industry there is less focus on truth and providing adequate care. Money has swayed research, and dubious statistics featuring a conniving emphasis on *cumulative* data make it appear as if HIV infections never significantly decrease from year to year,[187] thus maintaining public sympathy. If the Perth Group and Lance hypotheses are correct, a successful vaccine could never be developed because the problem is not the production of effective antibodies, but why a body has to produce so many to threats it could ordinarily deal with at the innate level.

What I would propose is to examine just how vitamin D deficient *or insensitive* HIV/AIDS patients are compared to the general global population, why a difference may be so, and whether repletion could reduce the likelihood of testing positive and developing AIDS-defining – or other – diseases. Should the prevailing opinion crumble, we could see the pharmaceutical industry held accountable for playing a subservient role in worldwide autogenocide. Viral immune deficiency hypotheses for other animals might also be called into question.

I would like to say that this could happen soon but I don't see an end in sight. The final bell could be decades away and the prizes may be retained by the orthodox scientists who could simply declare, by conscious or unconscious sleight of hand, that they eventually eradicated HIV-produced AIDS.

As a side point, it may be worth looking into the validity of the hepatitis C hypothesis, for which there also exists no vaccine. Testing HCV+ could solely be indicative of significant liver damage via multiple reasons.

Interview: Joan Shenton

Joan Shenton is the founder and administrator of the Immunity Resource Foundation, a charity whose primary aim is to disseminate information challenging the HIV/AIDS hypothesis. Her résumé as an award-winning television producer with Meditel Productions includes documentaries that challenge the cholesterol hypothesis, as well as HIV/AIDS. Though not a medical expert, her frontline experiences qualify her as an excellent proxy for this subject. She released the film Positively False: Birth of a Heresy *in 2011.*

From your observations in sub-Saharan Africa, how important a role does good nutrition and sanitation play in preventing HIV positivity and enhancing the health outcomes of the poor in this region?

I would say it's absolutely crucial because I believe poor nutrition leads to what used to be called slim disease – cachexia – which is when you get thinner and thinner, and your body races to protect itself by producing lots of antibodies which can make you test HIV+. It's actually malnutrition that causes HIV positivity.

Sanitation is absolutely crucial. My Meditel team filmed a pool in a low area of Kyotera in Uganda where children collect water, and discovered that all of a cesspit drains into it, and animals feed from it. Children there will have parasitic assaults almost from birth, so their immune systems are going to be eroded. Their ability to absorb nutrients is going to be desperately affected.

Then there's malaria which can leave you deeply

immune-compromised if you contract it seven times before the age of seven, or even just once. Orthodox medical papers even state that it leads to sticky cells which flag up as HIV; the same with tuberculosis.

Is TB endemic there and is this a common cause of false positives?

Yes. One of the things that happened in the early days of AIDS was that only extrapulmonary TB qualified as an AIDS-defining condition, but then suddenly the Centers for Disease Control and Prevention decided to add pulmonary TB. The TB specialists I then spoke to were concerned that everyone with TB would be classed as AIDS patients, and this was indeed the problem for some of them who found that when their patients were diagnosed with AIDS, they were removed from TB wards, put into AIDS ones and given antiviral drugs. A lot of those people were no longer under the care of a TB specialist and probably were not getting the right TB medication. I remember Dr. Martin Okot-Nwang really bravely stood out and voiced his concern because all the money coming into his hospital in Kampala was allocated for AIDS. He was losing his wards, his patients, his funding.

Have you ever come across cases where HIV+ people lost their status upon improving their health, or regardless remained healthy while still testing positive?

I've known very few cases of seroreversion – which means losing HIV. I did hear about the nine women in the famous prostitute study in Nairobi who tested positive and then lost it, and I remember Peter Duesberg telling me that if they were well looked after over a period of time, got good nutrition and improved their health in other ways, then it is possible they will lose it.

Personally, I haven't known many people who have had it and lost it. Most who have tested positive have remained so, but many are healthy. I can't give you numbers but in all the conferences I attend I see long-term survivors; people from the early 1980s who didn't take AZT.

How destructive has AZT and other antiretroviral treatments been on HIV/AIDS patients?

There was a whole generation of young gay men and some women from that era who took high dose AZT (2-3000 mg a day) and none of them survived. None of them. After that, protease inhibitors were developed and cocktails of these (HAART) include some nucleoside analogue drugs which are like AZT, but in very small amounts.

My take on all of this, from talking to doctors at the last Rethinking AIDS conference in Vienna who support the dissident debate, is that protease inhibitors are actually useful because they're antimicrobial, antiseptic and anti-inflammatory. All of those properties could be very useful to someone in an inflammatory state who's struggling to survive because their immune system is so eroded.

The horrific thing is that orthodox doctors prescribe these drugs because they think they battle a virus, so they prescribe them for life. Not even cancer chemotherapy is prescribed for life. So people in a very vulnerable health situation are taking these massive doses of protease inhibitor cocktails and suffering some extremely serious side effects such as heart attacks, lipid shifting in the body with massive things called camel hump, Crix belly (irregular fat accumulation), facial disfigurement requiring extensive plastic surgery. Death.

Have many thrived on these drugs?
Those who have taken protease inhibitors for short periods of time and then stopped – and I know some – have done well. In fact some of them have never gone back to them because their critical phase was damped down.

Have clean needle programmes been effective in curbing the HIV/AIDS epidemic?
It's nothing to do with clean needles. I have to quote Duesberg: 'It's not the clean needle, it's what goes through the needle that kills you.' He, of course, believes in the toxic theory of AIDS which covers intravenous drug users, including haemophiliacs who have to inject factor VIII daily. These are people that are in fact dying because of the assault on their body due to what's going through the needle.

Are AIDS Rethinkers encountering more or less hostility these days?
There was a period in the early Nineties when the Amsterdam Alternative AIDS Conference took place where we thought things were going to change as that had a lot of support from orthodox scientists. But from then on it's gone downhill really; we are ignored.

However, only very recently at our dissident conference in Vienna the media was actually interested rather than expectantly abusive and dismissive. We had a press conference which a great many journalists attended, and the Austrian Press Association issued a press release which could've been written by us. We were absolutely amazed! Secondly, a worldwide network called Russia Today decided they would interview a dissident a day and that was amazing too. Medics, professors, and doctors from our camp were interviewed and I was lucky enough to be included because I founded the Immunity Resource Foundation. So, yes, these days things are beginning to shift a tiny bit but, of course, how long did it take Galileo to be pardoned by the Catholic Church? Three hundred and fifty years! I think another generation of scientists, medics and medical students will have to carry this onward.

Which alternative hypothesis makes more sense to you personally: Peter Duesberg's or the Perth Group's, and could you explain why you feel this way?

When I first started looking into this in 1986 I went through a sort of course in molecular biology with Peter Duesberg to make our four related *Dispatches* (TV series) programmes for Channel 4. I was, of course, very interested in the theory that HIV was a dormant passenger retrovirus.

Then I heard about the Perth Group's work which agreed with Duesberg that HIV doesn't cause AIDS, *but* disputed its isolation, saying that what we're seeing is an antibody response which is being called specific to certain proteins that are called specific to HIV. So, I discussed these points every evening for many many months with the late Huw Christie who edited *Continuum* magazine – as Meditel shared offices with *Continuum* – and little by little, I *genuinely* found the Perth Group's point more persuasive. I've heard Peter Duesberg defend his theory, of course, that HIV exists and can be cloned, but I am less persuaded by that today.

How reliable are HIV tests and can you explain why this is so?

There's no gold standard for HIV test kits. Vaccines for flu, whooping cough, many things, can give you a profile that makes you test positive. You can take huge amounts of medicinal or recreational drugs tonight, go dancing all night, not eat, not sleep, and if you have a test early next morning you might test positive.

Back in the late Nineties we thought we could produce a one hour programme for World AIDS Day in which we were going to show the results of our tests that Channel 4 funded.

Our first lot of tests involved thirty-nine blood samples from people who were possibly considered to be in an inflammatory condition. We did this because Dr. Philip Mortimer at the Public Health Laboratories – our government laboratories – expressed great concern over how specific tests had been for over a decade, which made us want to examine where there would be cross-reactions. So we put these first samples through three different commercial test kits for processing in a virology lab in University College London. The Robens Institute at Surrey University handled the study.

We did two runs with the three kits and the first two test kits results were quite similar. The third test kit results were delayed for some reason, but when they came, nineteen of those which had tested negative on the first two test kits, tested indeterminate. Nineteen is quite a large figure. And in those nineteen was the blood of patients with TB, malaria and lupus. One of those people tested was a young man who tested positive six times in our tests, because it's two runs, three kits. At two leading teaching hospitals in London we took him to he tested negative both times.

In another test we took four anonymous blood samples from people with high gamma globulins (proteins) – perhaps with conditions like rheumatoid arthritis or lupus – that were provided by the protein reference laboratory at St. George's Hospital, Tooting, and one of the four definitely tested positive with no AIDS-defining diseases, or so I'm told.

The other eye-opening investigation concerned the Western Blot. This is commonly used around the world as a confirmatory test following an ELISA (enzyme-linked immunosorbent assay), but no longer in England. Dr. Mortimer had been extremely worried about the specificity of the Western Blot, which led him to recommend a double ELISA test for England and Wales instead; meaning that if you tested indeterminate on an initial ELISA you would then have another. He felt this gave a more reliable picture. Scotland, however, stuck with the original recommendation and in America at that time I believe it was illegal to call anyone positive without a Western Blot.

Anyway, we had sixteen further blood samples which we tested in England on ELISA then sent to Scotland for Western Blot. Of those sixteen, twelve were negative in London, six of those – that's 50% – were positive or indeterminate in Scotland. That is hugely significant in this tiny test. Back then there were a hundred and eighty thousand people in the UK in total who were HIV+ by Western Blot confirmation. It just makes you wonder how many of them then were false positive, and if HIV hasn't been isolated, then, of course, there are no true positives.

Is HIV common in haemophiliacs?
It is, but it's dose-related. Meditel did a lot of investigation on related studies and we discovered that an antibody-positive test result is found when a person takes high doses of factor VIII over a long period of time. The more severe your haemophilia, the more drugs you take, the more likely you are to test positive. The drugs are in fact an assault to the immune system because you're being injected with foreign proteins and your body's

reacting against them all the time. Age is also a factor.

Given how accepted the classic HIV/AIDS hypothesis is do you really believe majority public opinion will ever be swayed?
Yes, of course I do. I believe in the drip, drip effect. The Berlin Wall came down, who would've believed that? I'm very hopeful because the knowledge is now out, you know? The problem is censorship and peer review because of the vested financial interests, which brings me to Peter Duesberg's article co-written with Joshua Nicholson, David Rasnick, Christian Fiala and Henry Bauer, published in a journal called *Medical Hypotheses* and appearing on the Elsevier website.

Their article refuted one by Dr. Pride Chigwedere that estimated hundreds of thousands of deaths in South Africa due to President Mbeki and his panel of dissident experts – including Duesberg – advising against expensive and toxic antivirals in favour of improved nutrition and sanitation for better health. Mbeki and his panel were, of course, heavily criticised worldwide, and he was vilified in the most unjust way that nearly cost him his presidency. Anyway, this paper by Duesberg et al. criticised that estimation because the population of South Africa actually *doubled* in the period mentioned by Chigwedere; literally doubled. So what happened next? The editor of *Medical Hypotheses* was fired by Elsevier and Peter Duesberg was investigated for about a year by the head of California, Berkeley University. Duesberg was judged anonymously by so-called peers who were biased against him, but common sense prevailed and in July this year he was cleared by someone higher-up with wisdom who thought the charges were ridiculous. That is the most terrifying form of censorship.

The last thing is that the results of those tests Meditel

had done, that I mentioned earlier, were, of course, meant for a one hour programme on Channel 4. At that time there were top-level changes at Channel 4 so despite the eighteen thousand pounds we were given by them for our research, our slot was cancelled for World AIDS Day. This was in the late Nineties. We were then shifted across to the news programme so that we might just do an eight minute segment instead, which was impossible really, but Huw Christie and I produced something solid anyway concerning the World AIDS Conference in Geneva and we mentioned all the Perth Group's doubts. However, the night before transmission it was pulled.

Christine Maggiore's death is cited as an exoneration of the prevailing view. As a friend of hers what's your opinion on this?
I saw Christine at the Ekaterinburg International Conference on AIDS in 2008 and she was in good health. She was there with her son and mother and gave a magnificent speech... I was totally shocked because there was no indication she could die so soon, just a few months later of pneumonia, apparently; despite antibiotic treatment. Of course, it was linked to her so-called HIV status which appeared to fluctuate between positive and negative. Her death was due to some immune condition but I would certainly not say she died of AIDS. There are many people who die young of pneumonia and I happened to know one personally.

In 2000 you interviewed then South African President Thabo Mbeki who questioned the HIV hypothesis for which he was subsequently blamed for an explosion of AIDS deaths. What is the defence of Rethinkers on this?
I was shocked and appalled at the way he was treated, and

how the pharmaceutical industry clamped down on his very commendable effort to invite some scientists out for a discussion and to carry out some tests.

At the time then President Clinton was flying around the world pushing for reduced price antivirals and Nelson Mandela had set up his foundation. Both of those actions were based on the infectious hypothesis, so if you're against Clinton and Mandela you don't survive.

You've lent support to doubters of the cholesterol hypothesis, do you still stand by them?
Of course, even though lots of things have moved on since the Eighties where I spent a long time looking into it with Dr. James Le Fanu, and made three documentaries about it for Channel 4 and TSW (Television South West). Back then we had challenged the idea of changing the national diet in order to bring down peoples' cholesterol as Dr. Le Fanu believed that that was a very dangerous thing to do. For this we were, of course, branded heretical, so the health education authority clamped down on TSW and tried to prevent us from transmitting our film. My commissioning editor at Channel 4 also refused to put it out, so I approached the IBA (Independent Broadcasting Authority) who liked it and helped us air it. Those were the days when you could appeal to higher bodies.

The point I remember Dr. Le Fanu stating was that we need cholesterol, it's absolutely crucial to us. To bring the whole of the country down by a change of diet in an evangelical way would bring a lot of people too low which would be catastrophic. What you must do is treat the top quintile – as he used to put it – of the population that has very high familial hypercholesterolaemia.

You can visit the Immunity Resource Foundation at

immunity.org.uk

8. Approaching Repletion

Walk into any health food shop or pharmacy and you should find vitamin D with ease, however, the form offered could be inferior.

While natural vitamin D3 (cholecalciferol) is becoming easier to find, plant-based vitamin D2 (ergocalciferol) is still visible on some shelves. It is also the form commonly prescribed. Should your bottle or packet not state the form, you can almost guarantee that it is D2.

D2's reign was due to its historical profitability. It was once under patent and had been marketed effectively by pharmaceutical companies. Increasing awareness of D3, however, has made the industry realise that D2's days are numbered; that to ignore D3 is to bypass sustained revenue. D3's lower cost doesn't equate to lower quality as it is at least equal, if not superior, to D2.[250][251] In being natural to us it is also certain to be less toxic.

D2 is deemed vegan-friendly since D3 is often taken from sheep lanolin – off a sheep's coat – and purified.[252] Thus the latter product is suitable for highly observant Jews, Muslims and select vegetarians via halal, kosher or gelatin-free preparations.

My brother's osteomalacia and seizures disappeared not long after the initiation of a month-long course of 50,000 IU per day in D2 form. However, this and a subsequent lower maintenance dose did not raise him above 50 nmol/L (20 ng/mL). It was upon debating with his consultant that I managed to port him over to D3, which eventually optimised his level following dose adjustments. Prior to the changeover high dose D2 had just become impossible to source anyway.

An initial misfortune was that the D3 was only available in quick-expiring syrup form. Furthermore, it could only be obtained through hospital pharmacies since it was classed as unlicensed medicine, likely due to "not enough commercial interest".[253] A few years later, however, 20,000 IU D3 capsules came onto the market which are GP prescribable; though doctors remain free to elongate the dose to the point of being worthless, for example, once-monthly to average 700 IU daily.

Physiological (frequently referred to in this book as "high"), normal, doses of D3 can also be purchased without prescription through a number of reputable sources. If buying from overseas, even the total with airmail could be cheaper than a payable NHS prescription. Physiological D2 doses cannot be purchased freely, which perhaps serves as a red light concerning their long-term safety.

Some believe that gelcaps – aka softgels – are better absorbed than tablets, but the powder capsules I and my brother have taken serve us fine. Young children may prefer liquid drops, while injectable vitamin D could ensure compliance in the isolated elderly. Oral spray or transdermal cream should also prove attractive to those averse to pills.

For those with vitamin D conversion issues, such as seen in kidney disease, active form (calcitriol: 1,25D) itself is prescribed. Calcitriol is a prescription-only drug given under physician guidance as it can easily invoke toxicity, even if tuned to be tolerable.[254] If you don't have conversion issues it is best to let the body regulate activation from acquired reserves as this is the natural and safe way.

Due to the belief that vitamin D can be bettered – made safe, perhaps more effective, or both – research is continuing into vitamin D analogues;[255] clones, which is what I believe statins unknowingly are. This is laudable if you don't believe that the patentability of such products is a driving factor. D3 cannot be patented and D2 cannot be patented again, so the pharmaceutical industry is highly eager to find the next goldmine.

Proof that analogues could demote D3 is a paper outlining the positives of the D3 analogue elocalcitol. The drug was shelved because it did not meet specific criteria for treating an overactive bladder, though it had a clear impact on enlarged prostates – compared to existing treatments – and prostatitis.[256] Analogues are currently employed for conditions like psoriasis,[255] so it's clear that as they become more successful the impetus to reluctantly champion the cheap will diminish.

Though there are many scientists calling for extensive research to clarify the efficacy and safety of D3 itself, the mechanics of peer review – a system where fellow scientists critique work before it is able to be published – needs looking at because it doesn't always weed out, for example, reviewers likely to favour submissions promoting analogues due to pharmaceutical ties. An article concerning another topic demonstrates that this problem isn't restricted to medicine.[257] Only when we have bilateral disclosures of conflicts of interest can we expect a fair analysis of the original versus the analogues. Wholesale adoption of open peer review will facilitate that.

The rule concerning dose is one size *doesn't* fit all. But for the majority of adults anything less than several thousand units daily is almost guaranteed to be worthless.

The 400 IU recommendation will not replete deficient adults.

Before starting supplementation you may want to test your vitamin D level first. Virtually all physicians correctly interpret a request as for the 25OHD (reserve) level, however, anecdotally, a minority look at 1,25D which is erroneous to measure since this can remain normal or even elevated in a person showing evident signs of deficiency due to frantic conversion of limited reserves. Therefore, it is important to ensure that you get a 25OHD test, which tallies with oral intake and/or sun exposure. A 1,25D test is useful for diagnosing a kidney problem which often manifests as low extracellular (outside organ) 1,25D.[258] It doesn't really measure intracellular (within organ) levels which should be lacking if reserves are.

If your 25OHD level falls between 125-250 nmol/L (50-100 ng/mL)[9] you need do nothing. However, if you know you're not getting enough sunlight or oral intake you should re-test through another lab. Searching for 'vitamin d home test kit' in a local web search engine should return results for finger-prick testing products that can be posted back to a lab for analysis. This may be the only feasible option for those unable to attend a clinic or are denied a test on public health services because their doctor deems it unnecessary. In my experience, I have found testing on the NHS reliable; results correlate with my behaviour and other health markers.

If your level is considerably below recommended, a stock approach is to take 5000 IU daily for three months then get retested. If you wish, you may take higher doses less frequently to achieve the same dosage, e.g. 20,000 IU every four days. The closer you are to the recommended level to begin with you may only need 1-2000 IU daily. Over time you might have to adjust your dosage a little after hitting optimal which is why blind consumption isn't advisable, particularly as there are rare, but nonetheless existent cases of supplements containing too much vitamin D.[259]

I believe it is not essential, though, to have your vitamin D level checked first as most of us are insufficient if not fully deficient, so you can begin with 5000 IU for three months. I highly doubt anyone will reach toxic levels of possibly more than 250 nmol/L (100 ng/mL), unless there is a manufacturing error. At minimum you should test annually, as I and my brother do.

The issue is not how much to take but how much your body requires. Genetics, weight, current health, skin colour and access to sufficient UVB are all variables that work for or against you; therefore *your* requirement is not necessarily going to match mine. Under the sun thirty minutes daily around noon might be adequate for a slim white person while an obese black person should consider at least double that. Speaking of weight, loss of it in those who need to – at least amongst women – results in previously fat-trapped vitamin D entering the circulation,[260] which in turn regulates the hormone leptin[261] to help sustain a better figure.[262] If you take oral steroids for a health condition, you should consider that this too might be worsening a deficiency.[263]

Supplement quality is another factor. Some may contain less vitamin D than labelled,[264] so if you can sustain an optimal level through a certain dosage of brand x, it might be in your interest to continue with that brand to avoid false dosage adjustment. But don't let price colour your judgement as bargains can be reliable.

For severely deficient people stoss therapy – supraphysiological (very high) doses over a short period, as applied to my brother – can quickly raise the vitamin D status. This is safe and even desirable as it yanks someone out of deficiency whose health may already be compromised.[265] It is best done under the supervision of a doctor who you can debate with on dosage. I did not undertake stoss therapy so it therefore took me time to reach optimality since my 'starved' body prioritised using over storing, and I was working out my average requirement.

UVB-prioritising sunbeds can be a good alternative to sunshine for producing vitamin D,[266] so long as they are used with a view to raising levels and not simply overzealous bronzing. This means that they shouldn't be the sole preserve of the pale-skinned. SAD light boxes as an alternative to sunbeds may be helpful, but I have heard very few positive anecdotal reports, perhaps because of their limited size. Regular full-body UVB exposure either way makes vitamin D testing less critical as you're letting your skin determine maximal dosage, which will always be the right amount given ample skin cholesterol, UVB intensity and time. Adhesive UV sensors currently only available in America through one company can help determine when to end a sunbathing session.[267]

Spray tanning should be avoided as this artificial layer is undoubtedly an obstacle to even incidental vitamin D production.

Getting your blood calcium checked is also advisable to ensure that you're not becoming toxic, as defined by a high level and undesirable new symptoms. But as in my experience, you will want doctor clarification if your blood level is only slightly above recommended and you don't feel unwell. The rise may just be temporary, as I found.

If your calcium level is consistently very high it is more likely because of an underlying sensitivity that needs to be addressed. Toxicity is more of a theoretical risk as there is little report of it in the medical literature, and even then it is unlikely to result in death or chronic health problems when reversed promptly.

If you have not yet been moved to obtain some vitamin D you probably want to hear a bit about the counter-arguments first. This is reasonable as *you* cannot make a valid decision without seeing both sides of the story.

Firstly, mainstream science is not against vitamin D in general as it is recognised as important to bone health. What is opposed is the free consumption of many thousands of units daily when not suffering from an apparent deficiency-related illness, or when you are thought to have little risk of developing one. But if sunlight gives thousands per day, either nature or our governments are wrong. Prevention is also better than cure and a balanced diet alongside regular blood testing should counter any adverse effects.

Sunlight, however, is the bane of dermatologists. The amount of sun protection products at your local pharmacy or supermarket is testament to their vision of eradicating skin cancer. While it is true that burning from overexposure increases melanoma risk, the irony is that UVB-blocking suncream deprives us of the very thing that can fight cancer, as shall be discussed in the penultimate chapter. If we were taught to love the sun from an early age, perhaps it could never be an enemy. For example, a pale-skinned sporadic sunbather, unlikely to be vitamin D replete, has more chance of burning than a naturally tanned white person who sunbathes regularly and has an optimal level; perhaps since childhood. As an additional note, if you are pale but replete through supplementation you might find tanning less perilous.

In Asians and blacks deadly melanomas commonly appear on pale body parts such as under the fingernails, palms or soles of the feet,[268] but if such people were vitamin D sufficient maybe the incidence or severity would decrease.

Since most of us can't get regular adequate sunlight we automatically please dermatologists by opting for supplements, but that doesn't mean that those who can access sunlight should ignore a free source. Controlled exposure is the key and there may be other benefits of sunlight not yet known about. The only people, though, who cannot really seek the sun over supplements are sufferers of rare diseases like xeroderma pigmentosum.[269] In this condition the skin is overly sensitive to UV light and unable to repair the damage caused by it.

A treatment called the Marshall Protocol, however, asserts that vitamin D consumption is bad for all of us, and that to treat certain illnesses it is better to become deficient and take low doses of antibiotics for a number of years.[270] Its architect Trevor Marshall – who uses the Dr. title despite not being an MD[271] – touts active vitamin D levels as important; emphasising that reserve levels lower because of illness[272] and that repletion prolongs sickness. It is true that the body will use up reserves when immunocompromised, but he ignores the fact that an optimal level truly helps people and acts as a buffer against illness in the first place. At present the protocol is not backed by peer-reviewed studies. The only evidence of its efficacy is computer modelling – which is prone to err – and anecdotes. However, one shouldn't be surprised if antibiotic use helps people to some degree.

Vitamin D advocates acknowledge that there are some

illnesses which require caution when approaching repletion. For example, tuberculosis – which took my maternal grandmother at a young age – requires slow introduction to prevent bleeding to death,[273] and sarcoidosis – which Marshall acquired – is known to cause overactivation of vitamin D,[274] inevitably leading to high blood calcium. This, then, is an instance where *elements* of the Marshall Protocol may bring benefit; but under any other circumstance vitamin D restriction is inadvisable. I, however, harbour concerns about the protocol's safety for any reason. One drug employed called Benicar is – as of writing – under investigation for potentially accelerating the death rate from heart disease;[275] and it is part of a class of drugs that may slightly increase cancer risk.[276]

While we should welcome an antagonistic view as it helps put the brakes on over-enthusiasm, Marshall's theory has too prominent an Achilles heel: the assertion that vitamin D reserves are *solely* immunosuppressive. If this were true, replete people would only get sick; they would be immunodeficient. Evidence demonstrates the contrary. Furthermore, there should be evidence that vitamin D harms AIDS patients. I cannot find any. Marshall, however, is less hostile towards sunlight but he hasn't shown how D3 in the skin could differ from the oral version, which comes from the same source material in another animal. To his credit, though, an upcoming – as of writing – external clinical trial will elucidate how two unsung vitamin D measurements (3 epi-25OHD3 and sulphated 25OHD3) are affected by supplementation.[277] We want to see eventually if there is a disparity in these when sunning or supplementing and what disadvantages that may present. At worst, I believe, we might learn that supplementation is only slightly less preferable.

I have debated with a couple of Marshall Protocol

advocates online and I found their arguments weak. Not only that, it is hard to gauge the protocol's success rate. Certainly, from anecdotal reports, not all patients tolerate the treatment or find benefit from it. Indeed, some even end up in an emergency room.[271] That said, I don't dissuade learning about it as you should be free to judge the theory. Just bear in mind that sun avoidance seems bizarre for sun-evolved humans.

Repletion in the non-hypersensitive should prevent the development of diseases that cause hypersensitivity. A good analogy is to ensure that a vacant property is appropriately locked externally to prevent a squatter breaking in who would internally secure the building to breaking point.

Hypersensitivity from infancy,[278] in some cases, may be due to adaptation to ancestral deficient levels. That is to say that biparental vitamin D deficiency could force a foetus to develop as 'fuel-efficient' in order to thrive on expected low reserves throughout life. The downside here is that anything but incidental sun exposure or low oral intake is now an unnatural threat. We need to ask ourselves this: do we want future generations to enjoy the sun? If yes, obtain enough vitamin D for their sake as well as yours.

Many who dismiss vitamin D so far are likely to have simply tried the recommended daily amount, or perhaps a little more, in D2 form, and found little effect. This is why there is currently little awe over the substance. Stronger campaigning and more evidence will change that but each day until then could prove deadly to the masses. The supplement industry has a good defence for vitamin D: 'we'll sell it, but you can get it for free.'

9. Influenza & Autoimmunity

If despite long-standing deficiency you manage to avoid major illness in your lifetime – perhaps thanks to decreased genetic susceptibility[279] or other beneficial factors – it is doubtful that you haven't been affected by the common cold or flu.

Prior to optimising my vitamin D level I suffered from either ailment as much as anybody else. On a few occasions I required a course or two of antibiotics to treat a subsequent bacterial infection[280] that would see me hacking up super glue-like phlegm and producing discharge from my eyes. Since then I have only had a cold twice; oddly during summer. Perhaps these were vitamin D-resistant strains? In any case their severity was low. As for influenza, I forget what that more irritating illness feels like. My brother and I haven't required antibiotics for half a decade now either. This could be seen as coincidental, but a randomised trial with Japanese schoolchildren showed that vitamin D might reduce the incidence of acquiring certain strains of flu.[281] A flaw in the study was that it did not measure vitamin D levels, so we do not know if at least some of those who caught the flu could've avoided it on a higher dose.

The reason vitamin D may work here is simply because it mass produces the virus and bacteria killer cathelicidin.[185] Thus vitamin D is an alternative to prescribed antibiotics. If you catch a cold or flu that does not easily shift while on an optimal vitamin D level you may just have acquired a resistant strain. I had taken

150,000 IU for three days on top of my regular amount during my second-last cold bout in order to speed up recovery – roughly following an obsolete Vitamin D Council recommendation that factored in body weight – but I found it didn't do anything, so there may be little point in "megadosing" for this reason. Regardless, you must never take such doses for more than just a few days, and ideally only if you're particularly poorly than impatient.

Lack of vitamin D likely explains why we commonly experience colds and flu in the winter as this is when we all expose the very minimum to the open air and sunlight is scarce. Because many of us are deficient year-round due to negligible UVB exposure, we can assume that lack of UV light as well as low temperatures during the final season greenlights bacterial and viral survival.[282] Their strength and our deficiency allows nature to 'clear out' the weak.

It is reasonable to be sceptical of vitamin D's cold and flu fighting benefits due to the failure of the often praised vitamin C,[283] but the proof is in the pudding: if your incidence of either ailment diminishes as your vitamin D level rises – while ensuring not to neglect necessary co-factors – you have all the proof you need. Randomised trials, where patients don't know what they're taking, are proving that the benefits of vitamin D are not simply due to the belief-based placebo effect.

Because lifeguards and regular sunbathers can achieve a vitamin D level of 250 nmol/L (100 ng/mL)[284] at the end of a good summer without toxicity, such people do not necessarily require winter supplementation to stave off illness as it could take a season or two before their levels drop enough, by which time the UVB-lacking seasons have passed and a new opportunity for replenishing arises. But if you're taking supplements than sunning in a guaranteed UVB hotspot there is no reason to cease winter intake as you want to maintain a desirable level than hope for an 'acceptable' interim low. Spring and summer sun seekers could just take 1-2000 IU daily during autumn and winter to reasonably plateau their impressive levels.

Since vitamin D strengthens innate immunity, it is possible, in some cases, that the annual flu jab given to at-risk groups such as asthmatics, diabetics and the elderly is a waste of time when given to the vitamin D replete. Vaccines work by aiming to stimulate the adaptive immune system to produce antibodies to dead or modified viruses that do not cause disease. These antibodies then provide protection from the harmful originals, destroying them immediately. Given that viruses can have many different strains, particular vaccines are employed depending on what is likely to affect the population at a given time. That said, if one's innate immune system is in prime condition the vaccine could be neutralised before antibodies can be produced. Regardless, as the flu can be deadly to the at-risk who are immunocompromised in some way, the jab is better money wasted than a life lost.

When the WHO (World Health Organisation) proclaimed a virulent swine flu pandemic in 2009 I was dismayed by the media's lack of scepticism. Here was a virus that frightened people into believing that even non-risk groups might require vaccination or treatment despite little evidence of remarkable infectivity, symptoms and death rate. An investigation by the *British Medical Journal* exonerated those who believed that financial conflicts of interest were instrumental in driving the hysteria, whether or not known by the WHO.[285] Even if the pandemic were a genuine concern, free or cheap vitamin D would not have been touted as the first line of defence. Car salespersons don't like selling bus tickets.

Think about why birds migrate to the warm south come winter, or why some animals hide and hibernate during this period, and you should conclude that it is advantageous to be out of an environment teeming with bacteria and viruses that could be detrimental after a poor summer.

As the human race was able to avoid extinction long before the discovery of penicillin in 1928, we can safely assume that for much of our history, before we became much civilised, that we weren't aching for an Alexander Fleming to come along. I still believe, though, that there is a role for prescribed antibiotics.

Another disease recently linked to a virus is the autoimmune disorder – a condition where the immune system attacks itself – MS (multiple sclerosis). Research suggests that EBV (Epstein-Barr virus), which can cause glandular fever, is related to developing the condition.[286] The reason for this perception is, because parts of the virus resemble myelin, a substance which protects neurons and ensures accurate communication between them, a misled immune system would attack this too.[287] The resultant destruction of myelin is akin to stripping the cable plastic off a landline phone; you can no longer communicate properly. When this happens with neurons you observe MS. The antibody cross-reactivity also, unsurprisingly, makes 'false' HIV positivity a likelihood in MS;[288] a potentially disastrous revelation if MS sufferers are diagnosed HIV+ first.

A presentation on MS and vitamin D by Dr. Sreeram

Ramagopalan highlights that EBV is a common, usually symptomless infection, and that those who suffer glandular fever as a result have a higher chance of developing MS, whereas those who have never been infected have virtually zero risk. Ramagopalan also suggests vitamin D supplementation as an alternative to a vaccine.[289] Since MS is more prevalent in certain parts of the world it is possible that geo-specific strains of EBV in the vitamin D deficient increase the likelihood of the disease.[290]

A 1998 paper suggests that in Scotland, where prevalence is highest, the indigenous white population may have a genetic susceptibility to the disease since they appear to retain their risk in other countries.[291] Fast forward over a decade later and more credence is being given to the theory.[292]

Disregarding genetics or unique strains that lead to MS, Scotland's poor levels of sunshine[293] compared to the rest of the UK are certainly detrimental to vitamin D production and favourable to viral resistance. EBV infection in youth may be a particular culprit since glandular fever is common among young people.[294] Interestingly, MS is less prevalent amongst African and Asian immigrants to the UK but we see the polar in their British-born offspring.[295] Logically, the reverse should be the case with Scottish migrants to sunnier climes; more incidence amongst them but less to their children, so long as sunlight isn't avoided pre and post birth.

Vitamin D may halt or provide respite from established MS[296] but it will not repair the damage done. Elevated EBV antibodies persist for life[297] which means so would the attacks on myelin until a real brake can be applied.

It is important to emphasise that sunlight itself, independent of vitamin D production, *may* be beneficial too.[298] We must also refrain from concreting MS as an autoimmune disorder – there is much yet to learn about it.

In another example, type 1 diabetes is thought to be triggered by rotavirus since its antibodies can destroy insulin-producing pancreatic cells.[299] Vitamin D obtained early in life appears to reduce the risk of developing this condition.[300] Type 2 diabetes, characterised by insulin resistance, is also speculated to be an autoimmune disorder, related to material from fat deposits in obesity;[301] a plausible claim given that the illness is common amongst the significantly overweight. The finding that type 2 diabetes is reversible in the newly diagnosed through a brief, intense, calorie-restricted diet[302] supports the view that excess fat is antagonistic. Furthermore, as mentioned in the previous chapter, weight loss should lead to trapped vitamin D reserves being freed, and this also tallies with staving off type 2 diabetes.[303] Heart disease too is typically seen as a disease of the overweight so it is no surprise that we see the two conditions accompany each other. Statins can even be offered to American diabetics regardless of cholesterol levels to prevent heart disease...[304]

Finland is not renowned for much sunshine so it's no surprise also that amongst its common illnesses it has the highest incidence of diabetes in the world.[305] This is a country that gradually reduced its recommended daily amount of vitamin D from 5000 IU over the last fifty years to 400 IU,[300] which is, of course, paltry.

As with MS, vitamin D does not present a cure for diabetes as that would require the restoration of pancreatic cells and a halt to autoimmune responses, so – as with most things – prevention is the key. I have read very few anecdotal accounts of vitamin D producing a sustained positive benefit on long-established diabetes. Testosterone therapy might bring benefits for men, though.[306] Either way, the limited effect of vitamin D in this area is not a reason to avoid it for other reasons. Better late than never.

In summary, regardless of whichever virus can trigger an autoimmune disorder, – and there are others – vitamin D could be the saviour if you act now and not tomorrow.

10. Popping Cancer

Perhaps the most exciting feature of vitamin D is its probable ability to fight a devastating illness that will affect more than one in three Britons[307] and a similar number worldwide. While there have been advances in how this disease is tackled, a cancer diagnosis, understandably, still arouses dread as treatments can be harsh and expensive, and the prognosis is not always good. That is not to say I have a quarrel with existing strategies, just that future therapeutics need to be economical on both the body and public purse.

Before we look at how vitamin D can have an effect it is important to understand first how cancer arises.

Ordinarily, the trillions of cells in our bodies have finite lifespans: they fulfil assigned roles, divide to produce replacements for themselves and die. But when a cell divides too much and stays alive it can form a lump called a tumour, which is classed as cancerous if its cells are able to spread to other parts of the body but benign if otherwise; the latter can be left untreated since its limited growth may not result in pressure against surrounding sensitive organs. In cancers like that of the blood (leukaemia) there is no tumour but still an overgrowth of cells. What causes an initial cell to rebel is complex since there appears to be no single cause. For example, though smoking is associated with lung cancer not all smokers will get it. Other contributory factors to cancer are advanced age, a weak immune system and bacteria and viruses.[308] This is interesting because it implies that vitamin D is an ultimate factor. So, does this mean that if you take vitamin D you can continue to smoke? Truthfully, optimising your level and smoking would be better than smoking alone, but quitting the habit full stop would do you and those around you more favours.

It is possible that viruses trigger more types of cancer than we currently believe. HPVs (human papillomaviruses) are associated with cervical cancer[309] and it would not be surprising if such viruses lose their bite in the vitamin D replete. The doctor of the late BBC journalist Ivan Noble who documented his brain cancer fight online may have been on to something when he explained, to begin with, that "...it was much more likely that [Ivan] had picked up a nasty infection on a recent reporting trip to West Africa."[310]

Almost all cancer preventive measures are not contentious. For example, government campaigns promoting a higher daily intake of fruit and veg[311] meet little resistance, so asking people to take another natural thing on top shouldn't elicit outrage, so long as the public are sold on the benefits. Ultimately, an irrefutable array of evidence should convince policy makers that much more than their half-hearted historical recommendation helps prevent and fight cancer.

What should get your blood boiling, though, is that synthetic clones of active vitamin D are being studied as cancer treatments;[312] their success could nix penny prevention. It is true that analogues could be safer than providing ordinary active vitamin D, but they seem unlikely to be more efficient than the reserve form we let our bodies activate of their own accord, barring any conversion issues. So how does it work then?

The wonderful thing about activated vitamin D is that it

retards tumour growth by inhibiting awry cell production and movement, deprives them of needed blood supplies, and induces apoptosis. That word's second p is silent but I prefer to vocalise it as the 'pop' onomatopoeically describes what it does to rogue cells. Active vitamin D can also convert cancer cells, if salvageable, into normal or near-normal ones[313] that are able to produce another healthy generation.

Apoptosis is a Greek word for programmed, natural, cell death. If we completely lacked it our fingers and toes would be clumped together as cells joining them in our early foetal stage would have remained, just like excess modelling material in a developing waxwork figure. In the same way, cancer thrives where there is no sculptor to remove it. Too much apoptosis, however, is also undesirable as this can cause an organ to waste away; this is distinct from necrosis in which cells die prematurely from external threats *and* are ineffectively cleared. Fortunately, a randomised trial in post-menopausal women has shown that vitamin D and calcium supplementation significantly reduces cancer risk with no reported harm to organs.[314] For people who currently have cancer, aiming all the way to 250 nmol/L (100 ng/mL) might be a better bet than accepting the lowest satisfactory level of 80 nmol/L (32 ng/mL) or thereabouts. Anything higher, however, may be toxic.[9] With cancer you could need a lot more vitamin D than you think and perhaps in conjunction with existing treatments if things have turned for the worse.[315]

Vitamin D deficiency could also explain why – according to recent American data – black women die more frequently of breast cancer than several other racial and ethnic groups.[316] While local healthcare inequalities could be factored in, the fact that blacks synthesise vitamin D more slowly is worthy of note. Interestingly, British black women suffer from aggressive breast cancer at a young age just as much as their American counterparts and treatment equality for the former doesn't present any improved survival rate.[317] This could be attributed to the fact that blacks suffer greater vitamin D deficiency at a younger age than whites. The conundrum, though, is why other, observed, non-white groups die less frequently than whites when we expect the opposite. The answer might be that the effectiveness of safe sun campaigns has essentially led white Americans to have vitamin D levels below brown-skinned people who do not follow a strict conservative dress code and who are stereotypically unconcerned about suncream. This would explain why there is some parity in the disease incidence rate of blacks and whites. Diet and genetic susceptibility could also play a part though. Women who would cover more of their body for cultural or religious reasons are not apparent in the statistics; certainly, those of almost obvious Hindu, Muslim or Sikh heritage haven't been included. British women *emigrated* from South Asia, though, have less incidence, with the least amongst Bangladeshi Muslims[318] who are noted fish eaters. Overall decreased incidence may be partly due to lacking genetic susceptibility and perhaps the consumption of potential anti-tumour ingredients such as turmeric;[319] not to mention some early incidental UVB exposure from their country of birth.

When it comes to skin cancer the results are as expected – whites have the highest death rate, followed respectively by browns and blacks.[320] Needless to say, lighter skin can burn easily and the outlook is less good if you are also vitamin D deficient, exacerbated through the use of UVB-blocking suncream. Cancer Research UK seem to have reluctantly acknowledged this latter fact by *slightly* modifying their long-standing militant stance on the dangers of the sun,[321] but a map showing the incidence of all cancers in the British Isles – revealing a shocking north-south disparity – suggests that their U-turn needs to be much more vigorous; Londoners are far less afflicted than sun-starved Scots.[322]

Just as sunburn increases melanoma risk, further external factors endanger other organs; for example, alcohol raises liver cancer risk.[323] But what affects areas such as the breast or prostate, aside from predisposition, is unclear. Though it's contentious to say, I wouldn't be surprised if the frequent covering of breasts with two layers of clothing has a negative effect. Similarly, testicles are external to the body to maintain a cooler temperature, something negated by hugging underwear and trousers.

Bringing things full circle, it appears that high HDL ("good" cholesterol) protects both men and non-obese pre-menopausal women from prostate and breast cancer respectively.[324] [325] Statins are not going to noticeably increase HDL, but you know what can, and it is that alone which may reduce the risk in non-obese post-menopausal women too.[326]

Should vitamin D emerge as *the* critical cancer fighter, the days of losing hair, weight and organs to survive should be numbered. Our animal friends could also rejoice if we address them. Perhaps the rampant life-endangering affliction of facial cancer in Tasmanian devils[327] is partly due to the nocturnal animals being forced into habitats that rob them of their usual daylight exposure when resting,[328] thanks to our ever-increasing territorial needs.[329] We, in effect, then, would be their cancer, and our extended longevity in one way or another is even a detriment to ourselves as we clash for limited natural resources.

It is important to remember that vitamin D optimisation doesn't guarantee against cancer but it should reduce your likelihood. Additionally, if established cancer has managed to destroy vitamin D receptors we have lost the lock for our key and this affects prognosis. Research into VDR restoration should help said patients, but with early repletion such a procedure may never need to be employed.

Interview: Prof. Bruce Hollis

Bruce W. Hollis is a professor of paediatrics, biochemistry and molecular biology at the Medical University of South Carolina where he also serves as director of paediatric nutritional sciences. He is considered one of the most prominent scientists in the field of vitamin D research. Additionally, Hollis is a panel member of GrassrootsHealth which aims to promote the benefits of vitamin D to the American public.

How reliable are vitamin D test kits and do you foresee the development of products that give users instant results?

I essentially developed what became the DiaSorin test which was conceptualised thirty years ago. I've been using it in my lab and it works fantastic. I think the seasoned British IDS-iSYS test also seems to do pretty well. The rest of them, though, are quite variable and that can be demonstrated by the problems one company – mainly – had in the Australian market this summer.

Instantaneous tests are not gonna happen. I've been involved in this for more than thirty-five years and know the complexities. Hoffmann-La Roche has had to withdraw products, Beckman Coulter, Abbott and Siemens haven't been able to figure it out, so a point-of-care test, in my estimation, is not possible.

Do you think that there are other natural substances which should be given as much attention as vitamin D for fighting cancer and other diseases?

Not that I know of. The reason being is that antioxidants like vitamin C and E have hazy functions. Vitamin D's role in controlling genes and preventing cancer is quite well-defined. If you look at it from a molecular and biochemical standpoint there's a huge amount of evidence to suggest that vitamin D would be effective even if we weren't looking at the epidemiological studies. Vitamin D controls a couple of thousand genes in one way or another, so it can't be ignored.

Vitamin A is retinoic acid and, of course, that has its actions at the gene as well, but we don't have any idea what compounds like vitamin C and E do at a molecular level. Just stating that such things are 'antioxidants', to me, means they're essentially nothing.

How much vitamin D do you take yourself and what benefits have you noticed on it?
I take 4000 IU a day and I've done it for about five years now. Before that I was getting severe respiratory infections to the point where I cancelled my travel in the winter; I refused to get on an airplane. Since I started taking vitamin D, however, I noticed that the frequency and, remarkably, the severity of these infections diminished to the point where I don't limit my travel any more.

It's also cleared up my periodontal disease, which, of course, almost everybody suffers from. When you go to a dentist they're always telling you to floss more, 'you have bleeding gums, they're detaching from your teeth', but that's largely nothing to do with calcium. This has to do with barrier function and infection, and that has totally been resolved in myself and many of my colleagues.

Do you support the use of mammograms for diagnosing breast cancer given that they emit

radiation which may contribute to the disease?
I'm not an expert enough to tell but I have a thirty-two-year-old, pregnant, stepdaughter who is undergoing breast cancer treatment and her tumour would not have been detected without an obstetrician feeling for lumps. A woman of that age is not gonna get a mammogram.

A friend whose sixty-year-old wife missed a mammogram one year consequently developed a substantial sized tumour, so if I was a woman with a family history and I was aged forty or more, I'd be getting a mammogram every year as opposed to declining it in fear of radiation causing an additional tumour. That's my feeling. My wife gets a mammogram every year.

How effectively is the vitamin D message getting through to the African-American and Hispanic communities over there?
When you want clinical trials sponsored by our government you have to include all races, unless you have a reason to exclude them. In this instance we, of course, don't because blacks are the worst affected.

That said, I don't get the feeling that minorities – especially African-Americans – are all that concerned about it. The people who take supplements to prevent illnesses are highly motivated in their well-being and I just don't get the feeling that that always happens in the minority population. Ignoring disparities in income and care received it still comes down to the fact that the darker your skin the worse your health outcomes. Some of my colleagues feel that that's because of the worsening vitamin D deficiencies in these populations. In looking at overall mortality – and this has been shown several times – the lower the vitamin D levels, the worse the mortality rates for cardiovascular and all-cause mortality.

Do all or most cancers have a common trigger, if so, what do you think this could be? There is a belief that it's a man-made disease.
I would say absolutely that the environment affects cancer rates. It would be that and a mixture of genetics. We're learning more about epigenetics and modifications in utero.

I'm not sure about food additives getting a bad rap though, as the truth is that they've prevented a lot of sickness. People used to consume aflatoxins which caused an incredible rate of hepatic [liver] tumours and these have basically been eliminated because of food preservatives, so it's a double-edged sword. People wanna go back to the day where we didn't have them, but we would end up revisiting things like aflatoxins which are highly carcinogenic.

Pharmaceutical companies are experimenting with analogues of vitamin D for cancer treatment. Is this purely for profit or could vitamin D be reasonably improved upon?
This has been looked at for about twenty years or longer now. About ten years ago LEO Laboratories in Europe was one of the leading investigators in this field and I remember talking then to the person leading the research for LEO, and they were running all sorts of clinical trials before they quit. The same happened with Hoffmann-La Roche in the States. I was involved more in the ways to measure these compounds than the actual clinical trials, but what was uniform was that the[ir] vitamin D compounds were *highly* hypercalcaemic. All of them. That's what LEO Labs told me. They said that some were less so than others, but in the end they all raised blood calcium to a dangerous level. They added that 'as far as we can tell, we can't get high enough tissue [active] levels

before actually killing the individual.' So the history of these highly potent analogues is of abject failure. There's only two success stories and they've been around for at least twenty years. One of them controls hyperparathyroidism in renal patients on dialysis while the other one by LEO Labs is used for the topical treatment of psoriasis. The drug companies are always looking for a magic bullet though, to treat some disease, some cancer, so I guess they still keep hoping for more successes.

How confident are you about vitamin D preventing and curing various types of cancer?
I don't believe that vitamin D will cure cancer. Once the cancer mutation has happened I think you're in trouble. But I firmly believe that vitamin D has a role in prevention. When you get breast or prostate cancer, by and large those tumours are hormone driven, meaning that if you supply them with sex hormones – though they didn't necessarily cause the tumour – they accelerate its growth; like gas on a fire. Vitamin D, from what we know, basically fights tumours. It drives cells into killing themselves or brings them under control so that the immune system has the time to find and destroy them, or enhance its protection against them.

Have you noticed any patterns of vitamin D-related illness in your family history, if so, did that ring any bells when you were first looking at vitamin D?
I've had a few relatives with colon cancer. I've been fortunate to not have anybody in our family develop multiple sclerosis. Of all the diseases related to vitamin D deficiency MS is the scariest. George Ebers there in England who's head of clinical neurology is the world's leader in MS therapy; he'd been powering a campaign this

year called Shine on Scotland which tried but failed to get the Scottish government to institute supplementation studies during pregnancy. I myself ran around with George back in 2004 trying to get Scottish neurologists to pay attention. MS isn't just a big problem in Scotland, though. Tasmania which is south of Australia but with the same population of people – meaning no genetic differences – has seven times the rate of MS compared to its neighbour. George and I think the environmental trigger is a lack of vitamin D.

I've based my whole career on this subject and when I give lectures I say I've been as guilty as anybody else because I was taught the same dated information going through school. I thought a 400 IU recommendation must've been the result of seriously concentrated research. What woke me up was a study by Reinhold Vieth over ten years ago in which he dosed people with up to 4000 IU for several months and all it did was push them into a truly acceptable vitamin D level. Robert Heaney published a paper a little after using even higher doses and found similar results. It makes you wonder then, that if we've known for thirty years that 20,000 IU can be made from the sun, how is 400 IU the requirement? That figure was basically pulled out of thin air and it's been accepted without question.

With government backing I and others went forth with further studies on higher intakes and we've never seen a single case of toxicity – ever; pregnant and lactating women were given up to 6000 IU per day. From then on awareness has continued to spread.

Is it possible that if the deficiency remains unaddressed through successive generations we could one day have a vitamin D-insensitive population?
If you look at how epigenetics works it could be possible.

I'm not saying definitely but it is possible.

As a GrassrootsHealth panel member are you satisfied with the progress the organisation is making, and could you tell me a bit about it?
They work very hard in trying to educate the public. When I look at public awareness in the States compared to where it was five years ago it's huge. Testing has gone up twentyfold, and that's partly driven by physicians but mainly through public opinion thanks to education by the media. Oprah Winfrey is able to reach millions of women who basically control the healthcare of their families, so she's helped in the success. Sales of vitamin D went up from around forty million dollars a year to at least five-hundred million. Supplements are cheap so that means there's a huge amount being taken by self-motivated individuals.

I was just in New Zealand and the contrast between them and us is incredible because their government doesn't fortify foods; their children actually have rickets. I was at a meeting where a physician showed documented cases of the disease but their health officials seemed unmoved. They don't even have supplements at meaningful doses, so going there to talk about the benefits of higher intakes on cardiovascular disease and infections was futile as they aren't even concerned about rickets.

Based on sales of vitamin D tests, I think that the Middle East and Europe are making progress though, thanks to increased awareness. Europe is, of course, not doing too well and you could blame a couple of guys there who control a lot of the public opinion – Paul Lips and Roger Bouillon; they're stuck twenty years in the past and don't see the benefits beyond bone health.

To me, the minimum serum level of vitamin D should

be 80 nmol/L (32 ng/mL). That's not the ideal, that's simply what it would take to adequately mineralise your skeleton. To obtain that level in a population you're gonna have to have intakes of at least 1500 IU a day. Think about what that means in relation to Scandinavia or New Zealand who are refusing to do any fortification. The problem has basically become political; if they've defined 25 nmol/L (10 ng/mL) as normal then there's no action to take, and that's the figure I've heard in England and elsewhere in Europe.

There's an incredible German study in which, first, blood was drawn from around six hundred people across all age ranges who had died recently either through suicide or accidents, – but no other pathologies – to test their vitamin D levels. Bone biopsies were then taken for very skilled histomorphology to find out if any of them had bone disease. You could never do this study on living people as, obviously, you can't take out bone samples from people who are alive. Anyway, when they plotted the osteoid volume and all these incredible parameters from the histomorphology it became clear that only when levels exceed 75 nmol/L (30 ng/mL) is there an absence of skeletal abnormalities. How that paper[330] can be ignored is beyond me. If you wanna be absolutely sure that people don't have those abnormalities you simply have to obtain that level.

The other funny thing is, you know how much harm there is in supplementing? None. There are no documented cases of toxicity with reasonable doses of vitamin D. The IOM (Institute of Medicine) here is gonna release a new recommendation soon, but like the last time I'm gonna pay more attention to the UL (upper limit of safe intake). In 1997 they said the UL was 2000 IU, but this was essentially based on a fraudulent study from 1984 which was carried out on a total of six patients in whom vitamin D levels were never even measured. It was stated that the patients developed hypercalciuria (excess calcium in the urine) and hypercalcaemia at a given dose, so a toxicologist took that paper and applied a mathematical formula to come up with the UL. I believe the data was fraudulent because it hasn't been reproduced, and since then literally thousands of patients have been given doses that are way higher with no reported toxicity.

On recommending a new UL the best data they can use is that published by Reinhold Vieth. His outpatients were given escalating doses of up to 40,000 IU and at that highest dose you couldn't detect any abnormalities. If you applied the toxicologist's mathematical formula here, assuming any toxicity occurred at that dose, you would end up with a UL exceeding 20,000 IU. If calculated more harshly it would be at least 10,000 IU. So I'm interested to see what data they use and what UL they reach. I would have no idea how they would come up with a reasonable UL if they ignore Vieth. There's just no data out there which suggests that vitamin D is harmful at the doses we're talking about. I'm eagerly awaiting the new report as much as anybody else.

Four days after this interview was conducted the IOM approved a mere tripling to 600 IU. The UL is now doubled to 4000 IU...

For more information about GrassrootsHealth visit grassrootshealth.net

11. A Brighter Future

While the road to global acceptance of revised vitamin D values will be rocky, the optimist in me is certain that the movement's vehicle won't breakdown irreparably halfway. And *when* we get there, solutions to the deficiency pandemic could be more innovative than blood testing and medicinal delivery mechanisms.

In public toilets you may have noticed blue illumination and wondered what this is for. This is UV light in order to deter injection drug abusers from finding a vein.[331] But what if UVB lighting were installed in designated places in hospitals to boost the vitamin D levels of synthesis-capable inpatients – who could be mobility impaired but are able to activate vitamin D – through controlled full-body exposure? This would not only remove one of possibly many pill bottles from a patient's cabinet but it also reduces the need for blood testing since toxicity is not a concern when letting the amount of cholesterol in the skin dictate production. Alternatively, like in the early 1900s, you could place people on hospital roofs for controlled exposure from the main source[332] when available.

When a patient is discharged, though, they would require, at the very minimum, one vitamin D test per year; this could be incorporated into recommended general health assessments. Testing which doesn't require the piercing of skin would be a fabulous innovation to attract the doctor-shy and squeamish. They may even give instant results like that for blood sugar. To retain freedom from probable trips to the pharmacy, an effective UVB bulb could be installed in the home bedroom beside a traditional one for use when naked and alone or with a partner; a timer could be set to programs that cater for combinations of skin colour and mass. Hotels could also install these for their guests, and perhaps airlines could utilise low emitting set-ups in aircraft for the daylight hours of long-haul flights; plus, if you're heading off somewhere warm, trips to the beach might be just what the doctor orders.

To ensure compliance in the elderly, who could struggle to produce vitamin D from UVB exposure, a select range of 'heavily' fortified food products would provide a largely covert way of approaching repletion. For example, many popular breakfast cereals already contain multiple vitamins, so high-median-level offshoots could be created to cater for a demographic that hates medicinal mediums and can't or won't respond well to UVB. Cautions would need to be printed on packaging to deter overeating, and consumption by those who replete by other methods, but the occasional mistake is unlikely to be harmful. Either way, testing is unavoidable to gauge whether one must increase or decrease intake.

For people who have any consequential deficiencies (e.g. vitamin B12) it would be an idea to produce combination formulations that adequately prevent or treat problems that arise from that so as to reduce the number of pills etc. a person takes. As of writing, there are vitamin D supplements that at least come with the co-factors required for it to work properly should your diet lack these.

Let's not forget pets too. If we are to keep domestic animals indoor-bound, their food would also benefit from fortification or complimenting with supplements at doses that cater for them, be it in capsule or drops form.

Another application for UV light has nothing to do with vitamin D and associated products but can compliment it. UVC can be used to sterilise an environment from bacteria and viruses,[333] which could make it a more attractive alternative to chemicals in ridding hospitals of superbugs like MRSA, or potentially toxic moulds in homes. In short, any enclosed environment may benefit from UVC exposure. As UVC – which doesn't strike Earth from the sun – might be damaging to ourselves and our pets,[334] any devices produced for domestic use or otherwise could need to incorporate limitation mechanisms or safety information. There already exists some commercial UVC sanitisers, so if the idea catches on properly, cleaning fluids we employ may only be useful for scent and freshness.

Similarly, UVB exposure on the skin and wounds might be an alternative to pre or post-surgery baths; this would be particularly useful in emergency scenarios to stave off infections. UV light may also be a suitable replacement for the hand wash gels staff and visitors are encouraged to use in hospitals.

Complimentary to substance abuse rehabilitation programmes, ensuring patients get enough vitamin D may help speed up recovery and prevent relapses.

While it seems a long shot that people worldwide will adopt permanent naturism, appreciation of the sun may spur new forms of fashion that skilfully bridge the gap between conservative and revealing. This doesn't necessarily mean the exposure of sexual organs but it would elicit debate about cultural principles. For example, would bare back shirts for men be cringeworthy?

Hopefully, embracing of the latest vitamin D science will allow these suggestions to come to fruition, not just for the novelty of it, but because they would decrease the need to think about repletion as humans once used to. We can only hope that that day comes sooner than later. Not least because there are cases where parents are wrongly brought to trial for injuring their babies where simple vitamin D deficiency was the culprit.[335]

Although these measures may weaken pharmaceutical companies, we will still need many medicines as sickness and death are ultimately inevitable; if from nothing else but accident or injury. But health services should not then struggle to provide costly treatments to fewer people. Animal testing may also be reduced.

Whatever your stance on global climate change is, it is not unlikely that it would bring benefits to currently cold and sunlight-deprived countries via reasons you can by now fathom.[336]

Veering away from vitamin D, it is important to note the benefits of *darkness* too. Logic would dictate that there is a good reason for the sun setting daily and the most obvious benefit is in providing a cue to sleep and recharge. The hormone melatonin – which is also available as a supplement – is produced when we are free from light, and, amongst other effects, promotes a good night's sleep which will undoubtedly benefit our immune systems.[337] Unfortunately, the invention of the light bulb and backlit electronics, not to mention late working or playing hours and intercontinental flights, have deprived many of melatonin production temporarily or chronically which no doubt adds to the problem vitamin D deficiency poses. Darkness, therefore, provides the yin to daylight's yang, and there may be more to it than just melatonin.

The final thing I want to discuss is the implication that vitamin D science has on something many people hold dear: religion. If you feel that this territory does not need to be addressed please close the book now. I have deliberately saved this topic for last as it may upset the sensitive and it is not directly relevant to the health benefits of vitamin D.

To truly accept vitamin D science you need to acknowledge – as you may have cottoned on – the theory of evolution, as popularised by Charles Darwin's work *On the Origin of Species*; that nothing is divinely created. If you are convinced that adaptation is why humans and other animals are naturally very pale in UVB-lacking northern climates you cannot deceive yourself. Our planet "...started off", to quote evolutionary biologist and atheist Richard Dawkins, as a "...fragment of dust spinning 'round the sun.",[338] and, indeed, many pagans worshipped the sun as a deity; without it there would be no life on Earth. Bacteria-like ancestors and our relatives in between would not have arisen – this book could not be. Evolutionary creationists may argue that evolution is a mechanism employed by God, but this presents two problems. First, the understanding of man being *directly* created is undermined, and second, one questions how the Creator arose; something omnipotent should be a product of evolution too, and if not, the Creator's creator ad infinitum must have originated from something small. Omnipotence from nothing is a hard leap to imagine, but something microscopic emerging and evolving from seemingly nothing is plausible. Evolution, then, is behind everything in one way or another. It even seems to reflect global religious history in an inverse fashion since monotheism demoted polytheism, and atheism should logically be the final successor.

No mainstream religions, or even cults, profess the importance of the sun. If any of them did we would see the devout frequently baring their skin instead of clinging on tight to scripture-defined modesty and garb. When I see middle-aged Muslim women covered from head to toe moving with a penguin-like gait I feel anger at the programming that is undoubtedly helping to rob them of their and their children's health. Modernised, free, Muslim women would agree that full-body covering simply enforces male chauvinism.

Vitamin D science unearths other errors in Abrahamic belief. To begin with, portrayals of Jesus Christ are typically problematic; he is often painted as – going by a web image search – having fair brown hair and pale skin, sometimes going as far as featuring blue eyes; but someone born in the Middle East to a woman indigenous to the region is unlikely to resemble a North European – unless you hedge that their father is human and white. If most cannot make a logical guess as to the appearance of Christ it is harder to believe he existed, let alone held any special status. Images of the Garden of Eden also seem anachronistic. If Adam and Eve were the first humans it would be expected that they were black rather than white, particularly considering that they were surrounded by large and exotic animals who could only suffer in a place with suboptimal UVB. Mount Arafat, believed by Muslims to be the place where Adam and Eve were reunited after their expulsion, is not a place given attention as an origin of human proliferation, but if it were, the black couple would've benefited from losing some skin colour immediately. Also, how can Israel be the Promised Land for all Jews when its white, and even black, citizens have been adapted for life in countries away from the Middle East? Wouldn't a Creator change the colour of non-Arab Jews on immediate entry? You only need to use your imagination to wonder which country comes after Australia in skin cancer incidence.

On a personal level, I find it hard to comprehend an afterlife for my autistic brother. A stock thought would be that his disability grants him automatic entry into heaven due to not being able to read a holy book or perceive right from wrong. What irks me, however, is that practice such as burqa wearing or – in the case of my mother – being an indoor-bound housewife likely diminishes an unborn child's ability to learn; the obligation of the pilgrimage is also robbed from anyone with untreated osteomalacia.

The disputed belief that an army of virgins await Muslim men (and women) in paradise is laughable; we assume their presentation is for intercourse but a method of procreation would be of little use to the dead in a land of the same; an orgasm is clearly an enticing *living* reward for conducting propagation. Our gender should be inconsequential in heaven, so the promise of many partners makes no sense. Even so, that reward is not everyone's idea of paradise. Furthermore, would people like my brother suddenly be able to learn and speak to avail of their gifts?

Islam critic Ibn Warraq points out in his book *Why I Am Not a Muslim* that "The Muslim rites of running between Arafat and Muzdalifah, and Muzdalifah and Mina had to be accomplished after sunset and before sunrise... a deliberate change introduced by Muhammad to suppress... association with the pagan solar rite.", and "Houtsma has suggested that the stoning [ritual] that took place in Mina was originally directed at the sun *demon* [emphasis added]... [who is] expelled, and his harsh rule comes to an end with the summer,".[339] My reason for singling out Islam specifically is simply familiarity, but I maintain that no current mainstream religion is really positive about the sun. Given that we are not aware of vitamin D deficiency as easily as thirst or hunger this is an unforgivable omission in scripture. The Islamic ritual of washing five times daily is also likely problematic by removing synthesised vitamin D from the skin.

I do not wish to entirely criticise religions as they unarguably present some fantastic cultural benefits, but that does not prove their truth. Religions survive partly because they are seen as ideals for living. Re-establishing them as flexible cultures would ensure that they continue to serve us sans the pernicious elements; God was most certainly a valid gap filler before science coloured our understanding. Though a godless world may seem bleak to some, good health and the ability to enjoy what life offers should prove an acceptable diversion from the unfounded worry of hellfire.

I'm going to leave the baton with Darwin, Dawkins and Warraq et al. as this is not a book about atheism. I have said enough that is off-message. I hope, however, that theists can conciliate sunlight with their faith and at least acknowledge that vitamin D science is an important man-made revelation. To me, appreciating the sun as a battery for evolution means one should only store a holy book as an ornament. I do not feel I am being disrespectful in pointing out a good argument. Religion presents other problems than ignorance of vitamin D and that is why we should question their value.

Bonus: New Dawn Fades – Does vitamin D deficiency help fuel the blues?

Late 1970s band Joy Division were perhaps one of the first musical groups meant to be defined as *"miserablists"*; meaning that they produced music and an image that was more of a logical heir to black American folk music than that from their generally "swinging" peers of the 1960s. From the 1980s onward, downbeat went wholesale and manifests today as genres that express melancholy in varying gradients. Though contemporary miserablism is far from an exclusive British product, what we export from the Isles appears to be the most iconic worldwide – almost to the point of caricature.

Going back to Joy Division and their city of Manchester in particular, I wouldn't be surprised if an element of the band's material was motivated by lack of sunlight. While this statement may make you choke on something you're eating, there is a logic to it. Consider the following paragraphs from a 1994 article by Jon Savage titled 'Good evening, we're Joy Division' which features in the band's 1997 *Heart and soul* boxset on London Records.

"Everyone says Joy Division's music is gloomy and heavy," says Bernard Sumner [guitarist]. "I often get asked why this is so. The only answer I can give is...why it was heavy for me...

["]The whole neighbourhood that I'd grown up in was completely decimated in the mid '60s. I was born and raised in Lower Broughton in Salford [Greater Manchester]: the River Irwell was about 100 yards away and it stank. At the end of our street was a huge chemical factory: where I used to live is just oil drums filled with chemicals.

"There was a huge sense of community where we lived. I remember the summer holidays when I was a kid: we could stay up late and play in the street, and 12 o'clock at night there would be old ladies outside the houses, talking to each other. I guess what happened in the '60s was that someone at the council decided that it wasn't very healthy, and something had to go, and unfortunately it was my neighbourhood that went. We were moved over the river into a towerblock. [sic] At the time I thought it was fantastic: now of course I realise it was an absolute disaster.

"...The place where I used to live, where I had my happiest memories, all that had gone... I realised then that I could never go back to that happiness. So there's this void. For me Joy Division was about the death of my community and my childhood. It was absolutely irretrievable."

What we see in this excerpt – if the interviewee is honest – is that, for at least one member, moving into a place that inhibited outdoor play affected their mood for various reasons, which pooled into a black fount for use in an artistic endeavour. Dr. David Grimes, who is also a Mancunian, has detailed the impact of the Industrial Revolution on health in his book *Vitamin D and Cholesterol: The importance of the sun*, which lends credence to Sumner's words.

In essence, then, I wonder if – whether coupled with other personal factors – a band making *sincere* dark music like

Joy Division could exist without members affected by significant sunlight deficiency, which, of course, leads to a dearth of vitamin D and possibly resultant mood disorders. In other words, with more sunlight exposure, could there have been more 'joy' in Joy Division? Their tragic, tall, frontman hung himself in his early twenties, and he had been suffering from epilepsy, an additional possible indicator of vitamin D deficiency.

This is not to say that dark music is necessarily by and for depressives, because – as with books and films – conflict engages everybody and can even raise one's mood. Furthermore, uplifting music is not out of the bounds of the unhappy who may want to mask their feelings, pep themselves up or be subservient to others. A happy song, however, can still have a dark heart, and vice versa; the feel of a melody can be subjective.

Miserablism – really a byword for a subset of indie music – isn't the only descendant of the blues, though. External rather than internal discordance exists as heavy metal which began to take full shape in the 1970s with Black Sabbath. And let's not forget all the expressive world music which pre-dates the pop format.

Do I predict, then, that vitamin D optimality will hinder the blues and its derivatives? Certainly not. Anguish cannot be wiped out, but the producer of that is then likely to be self-limiting sadness than long-standing depression. If art is often seen as a reflection of society we should heed the cue that darkness, sometimes, literally, just signifies a lack of light and nothing metaphorical.

Though miserablist music has no particular UK hub, it is interesting that Scotland's most recent visible names –

e.g. Susan Boyle, Travis – deliver a lot of the less saccharine stuff. There are counterexamples, of course, but in a place virtually devoid of sunshine would there be justification to not write 'Why Does It Always Rain on Me?' Wales, which produced the desolation-capturing Manic Street Preachers, had an economy which depended on many working underground, away from scant light in coal mines, only to be replaced by mass unemployment and the social maladies that fosters.

I don't expect artists to sing about vitamin D deficiency, but if they can't name a source of their pain an implicit allusion to a setting sun would do.

*Excerpt from 'Good evening, we're Joy Division'
used with permission of the author.

References

PMIDs can be entered at ncbi.nlm.nih.gov/pubmed/ for access to abstracts and full texts.

1. Awakening

[1] Bodnar LM, Catov JM, Simhan HN, Holick MF, Powers RW, Roberts JM. Maternal vitamin D deficiency increases the risk of preeclampsia. *J Clin Endocrinol Metab.* 2007 Sep;92(9):3517-22. **PMID: 17535985**

[2] Hardwick LL, Jones MR, Brautbar N, Lee DB. Magnesium absorption: mechanisms and the influence of vitamin D, calcium and phosphate. *J Nutr.* 1991 Jan;121(1):13-23. Review. **PMID: 1992050**

[3] Rayman MP, Bode P, Redman CW. Low selenium status is associated with the occurrence of the pregnancy disease preeclampsia in women from the United Kingdom. *Am J Obstet Gynecol.* 2003 Nov;189(5):1343-9. **PMID: 14634566**

[4] Hewison M. Vitamin D and innate immunity. *Curr Opin Investig Drugs.* 2008 May;9(5):485-90. Review. **PMID: 18465658**

[5] Forman JP, Giovannucci E, Holmes MD, Bischoff-Ferrari HA, Tworoger SS, Willett WC, Curhan GC. Plasma 25-hydroxyvitamin D levels and risk of incident hypertension. *Hypertension.* 2007 May;49(5):1063-9. **PMID: 17372031**

[6] Rothberg AD, Pettifor JM, Cohen DF, Sonnendecker EW, Ross FP. Maternal-infant vitamin D relationships during breast-feeding. *J Pediatr.* 1982 Oct;101(4):500-3. **PMID: 7119949**

[7] Inflammatory bowel disease: Treatment. Vitamin D Council. Last updated May 6, 2010. Retrieved July 16, 2011, from http://v.gd/YkI07F

[8] Richards JB, Valdes AM, Gardner JP, Paximadas D, Kimura M, Nessa A, Lu X, Surdulescu GL, Swaminathan R, Spector TD, Aviv A. Higher serum vitamin D concentrations are associated with longer leukocyte telomere length in women. *Am J Clin Nutr*. 2007 Nov;86(5):1420-5. **PMID: 17991655**

[9] Vitamin D, 25-Hydroxy Level. Legacy Laboratory Services. Last updated November 30, 2010. Retrieved July 16, 2011, from http://v.gd/cvczpT

[10] Vieth R. Vitamin D supplementation, 25-hydroxyvitamin D concentrations, and safety. *Am J Clin Nutr*. 1999 May;69(5):842-56. Review. **PMID: 10232622**

2. Skeletal Effects

[11] Mellanby, T. The part played by an "accessory factor" in the production of experimental rickets. A further demonstration of the part played by accessory food factors in the aetiology of rickets. *J Physiology* 1918; 52:11.

[12] Goldblatt H, Soames KM. A Study of Rats on a Normal Diet Irradiated daily by the Mercury Vapour Quartz Lamp or kept in Darkness. *Biochem J*. 1923;17(2):294-7. **PMID: 16743184**

[13] Wolf G. The discovery of vitamin D: the contribution of Adolf Windaus. *J Nutr*. 2004 Jun;134(6):1299-302. Erratum in: *J Nutr*. 2004 Aug;134(8):2015. **PMID: 15173387**

[14] Marcovitz PA, Tran HH, Franklin BA, O'Neill WW, Yerkey M, Boura J, Kleerekoper M, Dickinson CZ. Usefulness of

bone mineral density to predict significant coronary artery disease. *Am J Cardiol.* 2005 Oct 15;96(8):1059-63. **PMID: 16214438**

[15] Rogers MJ. Statins: lower lipids and better bones? *Nat Med.* 2000 Jan;6(1):21-3. **PMID: 10671078**

[16] Chairman's Report To Shareholders. Pfizer. 2009. Retrieved January 29, 2011, from http://v.gd/qzOVzj (PDF) see page 14.

[17] Pérez-Castrillón JL, Vega G, Abad L, Sanz A, Chaves J, Hernandez G, Dueñas A. Effects of Atorvastatin on vitamin D levels in patients with acute ischemic heart disease. *Am J Cardiol.* 2007 Apr 1;99(7):903-5. **PMID: 17398180**

[18] Bhatty SA, Shaikh NA, Irfan M, Kashif SM, Vaswani AS, Sumbhai A, Gunpat. Vitamin D deficiency in fibromyalgia. *J Pak Med Assoc.* 2010 Nov;60(11):949-51. **PMID: 21375201**

[19] Aishah AB, Foo YN. A retrospective study of serum calcium levels in a hospital population in Malaysia. *Med J Malaysia.* 1995 Sep;50(3):246-9. **PMID: 8926903**

[20] Sojka JE, Weaver CM. Magnesium supplementation and osteoporosis. *Nutr Rev.* 1995 Mar;53(3):71-4. Review. **PMID: 7770187**

[21] Payne ME, Anderson JJ, Steffens DC. Calcium and vitamin D intakes may be positively associated with brain lesions in depressed and nondepressed elders. *Nutr Res.* 2008 May;28(5):285-92. **PMID: 19083421**

[22] MacLaughlin J, Holick MF. Aging decreases the capacity of human skin to produce vitamin D3. *J Clin Invest.* 1985 Oct;76(4):1536-8. **PMID: 2997282**

[23] No to Fluoridation. ISIS Report 07/01/05. Retrieved January

29, 2011, from http://v.gd/qv2t80

[24] Chapter 7: The Extent of Water Fluoridation. One in a Million: the facts about water fluoridation. 2nd edition. The British Fluoridation Society. June 2004. Retrieved January 29, 2011, from http://v.gd/PTw4FQ

[25] Haguenauer D, Welch V, Shea B, Tugwell P, Wells G. Fluoride for treating postmenopausal osteoporosis. *Cochrane Database Syst Rev*. 2000;(4):CD002825. Review. **PMID: 11034769**

[26] Water in your home. Thames Water. Last updated May 28, 2011. Retrieved January 26, 2012, from http://v.gd/EdQVo0

[27] Fluoridation of water. (Figure 1). British Medical Association. January 12, 2010. Retrieved January 29, 2011, from http://v.gd/yH8xuJ

[28] Drinking water quality. Ref no: WQB0001. Dŵr Cymru. November 2006. Retrieved January 29, 2011, from http://v.gd/r6pry4

[29] Sahota O, Mundey MK, San P, Godber IM, Hosking DJ. Vitamin D insufficiency and the blunted PTH response in established osteoporosis: the role of magnesium deficiency. *Osteoporos Int*. 2006;17(7):1013-21. Erratum in: *Osteoporos Int*. 2006 Dec;17(12):1825-6. **PMID: 16596461**

[30] Eskandari F, Martinez PE, Torvik S, Phillips TM, Sternberg EM, Mistry S, Ronsaville D, Wesley R, Toomey C, Sebring NG, Reynolds JC, Blackman MR, Calis KA, Gold PW, Cizza G; Premenopausal, Osteoporosis Women, Alendronate, Depression (POWER) Study Group. Low bone mass in premenopausal women with depression. *Arch Intern Med*. 2007 Nov 26;167(21):2329-36. **PMID: 18039992**

[31] Shipowick CD, Moore CB, Corbett C, Bindler R. Vitamin D and depressive symptoms in women during the winter: a pilot study. *Appl Nurs Res*. 2009 Aug;22(3):221-5. **PMID: 19616172**

[32] Dupree K, Dobs A. Osteopenia and male hypogonadism. *Rev Urol*. 2004;6 Suppl 6:S30-4. **PMID: 16985910**

[33] Pilz S, Frisch S, Koertke H, Kuhn J, Dreier J, Obermayer-Pietsch B, Wehr E, Zittermann A. Effect of vitamin D supplementation on testosterone levels in men. *Horm Metab Res*. 2011 Mar;43(3):223-5. **PMID: 21154195**

3. Brain Development & Maintenance

[34] Lee DM, Tajar A, Ulubaev A, Pendleton N, O'Neill TW, O'Connor DB, Bartfai G, Boonen S, Bouillon R, Casanueva FF, Finn JD, Forti G, Giwercman A, Han TS, Huhtaniemi IT, Kula K, Lean ME, Punab M, Silman AJ, Vanderschueren D, Wu FC; EMAS study group. Association between 25-hydroxyvitamin D levels and cognitive performance in middle-aged and older European men. *J Neurol Neurosurg Psychiatry*. 2009 Jul;80(7):722-9. **PMID: 19460797**

[35] Cannell JJ. Autism and vitamin D. *Med Hypotheses*. 2008;70(4):750-9. **PMID: 17920208**

[36] Wakefield AJ, Murch SH, Anthony A, Linnell J, Casson DM, Malik M, Berelowitz M, Dhillon AP, Thomson MA, Harvey P, Valentine A, Davies SE, Walker-Smith JA. Ileal-lymphoid-nodular hyperplasia, non-specific colitis, and pervasive developmental disorder in children. *Lancet*. 1998 Feb 28;351(9103):637-41. Retraction in: *Lancet*. 2010 Feb 6;375(9713):445. Partial retraction in: Murch SH, Anthony A, Casson DH, Malik M, Berelowitz M, Dhillon AP,

Thomson MA, Valentine A, Davies SE, Walker-Smith JA. *Lancet.* 2004 Mar 6;363(9411):750. **PMID: 9500320**

[37] Bishop DV, Whitehouse AJ, Watt HJ, Line EA. Autism and diagnostic substitution: evidence from a study of adults with a history of developmental language disorder. *Dev Med Child Neurol.* 2008 May;50(5):341-5. **PMID: 18384386**

[38] A history of SunSmart media campaigns. SunSmart. Last updated November 28, 2010. Retrieved February 11, 2011, from http://v.gd/rffgFD

[39] Frequently Asked Questions About Thimerosal (Ethylmercury). Centers for Disease Control and Prevention (CDC). Last updated October 14, 2011. Retrieved January 26, 2012, from http://v.gd/oGWExm

[40] Tierney E, Bukelis I, Thompson RE, Ahmed K, Aneja A, Kratz L, Kelley RI. Abnormalities of cholesterol metabolism in autism spectrum disorders. *Am J Med Genet B Neuropsychiatr Genet.* 2006 Sep 5;141B(6):666-8. **PMID: 16874769**

[41] Aneja A, Tierney E. Autism: the role of cholesterol in treatment. *Int Rev Psychiatry.* 2008 Apr;20(2):165-70. Review. **PMID: 18386207**

[42] Dietschy JM, Turley SD. Cholesterol metabolism in the brain. *Curr Opin Lipidol.* 2001 Apr;12(2):105-12. Review. **PMID: 11264981**

[43] Garcion E, Wion-Barbot N, Montero-Menei CN, Berger F, Wion D. New clues about vitamin D functions in the nervous system. *Trends Endocrinol Metab.* 2002 Apr;13(3):100-5. Review. **PMID: 11893522**

[44] Ehlers S, Gillberg C. The epidemiology of Asperger syndrome. A total population study. *J Child Psychol*

Psychiatry. 1993 Nov;34(8):1327-50. **PMID: 8294522**

[45] Losem-Heinrichs E, Görg B, Schleicher A, Redecker C, Witte OW, Zilles K, Bidmon HJ. A combined treatment with 1alpha,25-dihydroxy-vitamin D3 and 17beta-estradiol reduces the expression of heat shock protein-32 (HSP-32) following cerebral cortical ischemia. *J Steroid Biochem Mol Biol*. 2004 May;89-90(1-5):371-4. **PMID: 15225803**

[46] Yang SH, Perez E, Cutright J, Liu R, He Z, Day AL, Simpkins JW. Testosterone increases neurotoxicity of glutamate in vitro and ischemia-reperfusion injury in an animal model. *J Appl Physiol*. 2002 Jan;92(1):195-201. **PMID: 11744660**

[47] Ingudomnukul E, Baron-Cohen S, Wheelwright S, Knickmeyer R. Elevated rates of testosterone-related disorders in women with autism spectrum conditions. *Horm Behav*. 2007 May;51(5):597-604. **PMID: 17462645**

[48] Aschner M, Ceccatelli S. Are neuropathological conditions relevant to ethylmercury exposure? *Neurotox Res*. 2010 Jul;18(1):59-68. **PMID: 19756911**

[49] Eyles DW, Feron F, Cui X, Kesby JP, Harms LH, Ko P, McGrath JJ, Burne TH. Developmental vitamin D deficiency causes abnormal brain development. *Psychoneuroendocrinology*. 2009 Dec;34 Suppl 1:S247-57. Review. **PMID: 19500914**

[50] Van Heest R, Jones S, Giacomantonio M. Rectal prolapse in autistic children. *J Pediatr Surg*. 2004 Apr;39(4):643-4. **PMID: 15065049**

[51] Takayama H, Takagi H, Larochelle WJ, Kapur RP, Merlino G. Ulcerative proctitis, rectal prolapse, and intestinal pseudo-obstruction in transgenic mice overexpressing hepatocyte growth factor/scatter factor. *Lab Invest*. 2001

Mar;81(3):297-305. **PMID: 11310823**

[52] Lim WC, Hanauer SB, Li YC. Mechanisms of disease: vitamin D and inflammatory bowel disease. *Nat Clin Pract Gastroenterol Hepatol*. 2005 Jul;2(7):308-15. Review. **PMID: 16265284**

[53] Whitelaw A, Jary S, Kmita G, Wroblewska J, Musialik-Swietlinska E, Mandera M, Hunt L, Carter M, Pople I. Randomized Trial of Drainage, Irrigation and Fibrinolytic Therapy for Premature Infants with Posthemorrhagic Ventricular Dilatation: Developmental Outcome at 2 years. *Pediatrics*. 2010 Apr;125(4):e852-8. **PMID: 20211949**

[54] Tuchman R, Rapin I. Epilepsy in autism. *Lancet Neurol*. 2002 Oct;1(6):352-8. Review. **PMID: 12849396**

[55] Karpova MN, Pankov OIu, Glebov RN, Dubur GIa, Germane SK, Klusha VE. [Anti-epileptic effect of the new calcium channel blocker IOS-1.1212]. *Biull Eksp Biol Med*. 1991 Oct;112(10):362-5. **PMID: 1804343**

[56] Bar-Or D, Gasiel Y. Calcium and calciferol antagonise effect of verapamil in atrial fibrillation. *Br Med J (Clin Res Ed)*. 1981 May 16;282(6276):1585-6. **PMID: 6786574**

[57] Nakken KO, Taubøll E. Bone loss associated with use of antiepileptic drugs. *Expert Opin Drug Saf*. 2010 Jul;9(4):561-71. Review. **PMID: 20201711**

[58] Holló A, Clemens Z, Kamondi A, Lakatos P, Szűcs A. Correction of vitamin D deficiency improves seizure control in epilepsy: A pilot study. *Epilepsy Behav*. 2012 Apr 11. **PMID: 22503468**

[59] Etminan M, Samii A, Brophy JM. Statin use and risk of epilepsy: a nested case-control study. *Neurology*. 2010 Oct 26;75(17):1496-500. **PMID: 20975051**

[60] Wilkins CH, Sheline YI, Roe CM, Birge SJ, Morris JC. Vitamin D deficiency is associated with low mood and worse cognitive performance in older adults. *Am J Geriatr Psychiatry*. 2006 Dec;14(12):1032-40. **PMID: 17138809**

[61] Cherniack EP, Troen BR, Florez HJ, Roos BA, Levis S. Some new food for thought: the role of vitamin D in the mental health of older adults. *Curr Psychiatry Rep*. 2009 Feb;11(1):12-9. Review. **PMID: 19187703**

[62] Buell JS, Dawson-Hughes B, Scott TM, Weiner DE, Dallal GE, Qui WQ, Bergethon P, Rosenberg IH, Folstein MF, Patz S, Bhadelia RA, Tucker KL. 25-Hydroxyvitamin D, dementia, and cerebrovascular pathology in elders receiving home services. *Neurology*. 2010 Jan 5;74(1):18-26. **PMID: 19940273**

[63] Evatt ML, Delong MR, Khazai N, Rosen A, Triche S, Tangpricha V. Prevalence of vitamin d insufficiency in patients with Parkinson disease and Alzheimer disease. *Arch Neurol*. 2008 Oct;65(10):1348-52. **PMID: 18852350**

[64] Munger KL, Zhang SM, O'Reilly E, Hernán MA, Olek MJ, Willett WC, Ascherio A. Vitamin D intake and incidence of multiple sclerosis. *Neurology*. 2004 Jan 13;62(1):60-5. **PMID: 14718698**

[65] Whitaker CH, Malchoff CD, Felice KJ. Treatable lower motor neuron disease due to vitamin D deficiency and secondary hyperparathyroidism. *Amyotroph Lateral Scler Other Motor Neuron Disord*. 2000 Sep;1(4):283-6. Review. **PMID: 11465022**

[66] Mackay-Sim A, Féron F, Eyles D, Burne T, McGrath J. Schizophrenia, vitamin D, and brain development. 2004. *Int Rev Neurobiol*. 2004;59:351-80. Review. **PMID: 15006495**

[67] López-Arrieta JM, Birks J. Nimodipine for primary

degenerative, mixed and vascular dementia. *Cochrane Database Syst Rev.* 2002;(3):CD000147. Review. **PMID: 12137606**

[68] Li Y, Hu X, Liu Y, Bao Y, An L. Nimodipine protects dopaminergic neurons against inflammation-mediated degeneration through inhibition of microglial activation. *Neuropharmacology.* 2009 Mar;56(3):580-9. **PMID: 19049811**

[69] Kapoor R, Davies M, Blaker PA, Hall SM, Smith KJ. Blockers of sodium and calcium entry protect axons from nitric oxide-mediated degeneration. *Ann Neurol.* 2003 Feb;53(2):174-80. **PMID: 12557283**

[70] Colom LV, Alexianu ME, Mosier DR, Smith RG, Appel SH. Amyotrophic lateral sclerosis immunoglobulins increase intracellular calcium in a motoneuron cell line. *Exp Neurol.* 1997 Aug;146(2):354-60. **PMID: 9270044**

[71] Yamada K, Kanba S, Ashikari I, Ohnishi K, Yagi G, Asai M. Nilvadipine is effective for chronic schizophrenia in a double-blind placebo-controlled study. *J Clin Psychopharmacol.* 1996 Dec;16(6):437-9. **PMID: 8959468**

[72] Umeda T, Mori H, Zheng H, Tomiyama T. Regulation of cholesterol efflux by amyloid beta secretion. *J Neurosci Res.* 2010 Jul;88(9):1985-94. **PMID: 20155813**

[73] Hyppönen E, Power C. Hypovitaminosis D in British adults at age 45 y: nationwide cohort study of dietary and lifestyle predictors. *Am J Clin Nutr.* 2007 Mar;85(3):860-8. **PMID: 17344510**

[74] Miyake Y, Sasaki S, Tanaka K, Hirota Y. Dairy food, calcium, and vitamin D intake in pregnancy and wheeze and eczema in infants. *Eur Respir J.* 2010 Jun;35(6):1228-34. **PMID: 19840962**

[75] Litonjua AA, Weiss ST. Is vitamin D deficiency to blame for the asthma epidemic? *J Allergy Clin Immunol.* 2007 Nov;120(5):1031-5. **PMID: 17919705**

4. Vegetable, Mineral & Animal

[76] Atkins diet boss: 'Eat less fat'. BBC News. Last updated January 19, 2004. Retrieved February 19, 2011, from http://v.gd/BZ2JGS

[77] List of articles by Dr. William Davis concerning the term 'wheat'. The Heart Scan Blog. Retrieved February 19, 2011, from http://v.gd/nUa2If

[78] Di Sabatino A, Corazza GR. Coeliac disease. *Lancet.* 2009 Apr 25;373(9673):1480-93. **PMID: 19394538**

[79] Kanai T, Takagi T, Masuhiro K, Nakamura M, Iwata M, Saji F. Serum vitamin K level and bone mineral density in post-menopausal women. *Int J Gynaecol Obstet.* 1997 Jan;56(1):25-30. **PMID: 9049691**

[80] Schurgers LJ, Teunissen KJ, Hamulyák K, Knapen MH, Vik H, Vermeer C. Vitamin K-containing dietary supplements: comparison of synthetic vitamin K1 and natto-derived menaquinone-7. *Blood.* 2007 Apr 15;109(8):3279-83. **PMID: 17158229**

[81] Schurgers LJ, Vermeer C. Determination of phylloquinone and menaquinones in food. Effect of food matrix on circulating vitamin K concentrations. *Haemostasis.* 2000 Nov-Dec;30(6):298-307. **PMID: 11356998**

[82] Cannell JJ, Vieth R, Willett W, Zasloff M, Hathcock JN, White JH, Tanumihardjo SA, Larson-Meyer DE, Bischoff-Ferrari HA, Lamberg-Allardt CJ, Lappe JM, Norman AW, Zittermann A, Whiting SJ, Grant WB, Hollis BW,

Giovannucci E. Cod liver oil, vitamin A toxicity, frequent respiratory infections, and the vitamin D deficiency epidemic. *Ann Otol Rhinol Laryngol.* 2008 Nov;117(11):864-70. Review. **PMID: 19102134**

[83] Why is a prescription needed for LOVAZA? Lovaza.com. Retrieved March 25, 2010, from http://v.gd/hb1ouE Retrieval as of February 19, 2011 does not display comparison with standard fish oil capsules.

[84] Wortsman J, Matsuoka LY, Chen TC, Lu Z, Holick MF. Decreased bioavailability of vitamin D in obesity. *Am J Clin Nutr.* 2000 Sep;72(3):690-3. Erratum in: *Am J Clin Nutr.* 2003 May;77(5):1342. **PMID: 10966885**

[85] Al-Elq AH, Sadat-Ali M, Al-Turki HA, Al-Mulhim FA, Al-Ali AK. Is there a relationship between body mass index and serum vitamin D levels? *Saudi Med J.* 2009 Dec;30(12):1542-6. **PMID: 19936417**

[86] Jackson RD, LaCroix AZ, Gass M, Wallace RB, Robbins J, Lewis CE, Bassford T, Beresford SA, Black HR, Blanchette P, Bonds DE, Brunner RL, Brzyski RG, Caan B, Cauley JA, Chlebowski RT, Cummings SR, Granek I, Hays J, Heiss G, Hendrix SL, Howard BV, Hsia J, Hubbell FA, Johnson KC, Judd H, Kotchen JM, Kuller LH, Langer RD, Lasser NL, Limacher MC, Ludlam S, Manson JE, Margolis KL, McGowan J, Ockene JK, O'Sullivan MJ, Phillips L, Prentice RL, Sarto GE, Stefanick ML, Van Horn L, Wactawski-Wende J, Whitlock E, Anderson GL, Assaf AR, Barad D; Women's Health Initiative Investigators. Calcium plus vitamin D supplementation and the risk of fractures. *N Engl J Med.* 2006 Feb 16;354(7):669-83. Erratum in: *N Engl J Med.* 2006 Mar 9;354(10):1102. **PMID: 16481635**

[87] Wysolmerski JJ. The evolutionary origins of maternal calcium and bone metabolism during lactation. *J Mammary*

Gland Biol Neoplasia. 2002 Jul;7(3):267-76. Review. **PMID: 12751891**

[88] Holick MF. Vitamin D: importance in the prevention of cancers, type 1 diabetes, heart disease, and osteoporosis. *Am J Clin Nutr*. 2004 Mar;79(3):362-71. Review. Erratum in: *Am J Clin Nutr*. 2004 May;79(5):890. **PMID: 14985208**

[89] Osteoporosis tigers back on prowl. BBC News. Last updated October 28, 2009. Retrieved February 19, 2011, from http://v.gd/ALSb2t

[90] Vitamin-D Phototherapy Frequently Asked Questions (FAQ). Solarc Systems Inc. Retrieved January 27, 2011, from http://v.gd/LwyFBL

[91] Gray MM, Sutter NB, Ostrander EA, Wayne RK. The IGF1 small dog haplotype is derived from Middle Eastern grey wolves. *BMC Biol*. 2010 Feb 24;8:16. **PMID: 20181231**

[92] Hyppönen E, Boucher BJ, Berry DJ, Power C. 25-hydroxyvitamin D, IGF-1, and metabolic syndrome at 45 years of age: a cross-sectional study in the 1958 British Birth Cohort. *Diabetes*. 2008 Feb;57(2):298-305. **PMID: 18003755**

[93] Driscoll CA, Menotti-Raymond M, Roca AL, Hupe K, Johnson WE, Geffen E, Harley EH, Delibes M, Pontier D, Kitchener AC, Yamaguchi N, O'brien SJ, Macdonald DW. The Near Eastern origin of cat domestication. *Science*. 2007 Jul 27;317(5837):519-23. **PMID: 17600185**

[94] McKenna MJ. Differences in vitamin D status between countries in young adults and the elderly. *Am J Med*. 1992 Jul;93(1):69-77. **PMID: 1385673**

[95] Meyer HE, Falch JA, O'Neill T, Tverdal A, Varlow J. Height and body mass index in Oslo, Norway, compared to other

regions of Europe: do they explain differences in the incidence of hip fracture? European Vertebral Osteoporosis Study Group. *Bone*. 1995 Oct;17(4):347-50. **PMID: 8573406**

[96] Slingerland LI, Fazilova VV, Plantinga EA, Kooistra HS, Beynen AC. Indoor confinement and physical inactivity rather than the proportion of dry food are risk factors in the development of feline type 2 diabetes mellitus. *Vet J.* 2009 Feb;179(2):247-53. **PMID: 17964833**

[97] Morris JG. Ineffective vitamin D synthesis in cats is reversed by an inhibitor of 7-dehydrocholestrol-delta7-reductase. *J Nutr*. 1999 Apr;129(4):903-8. **PMID: 10203568**

[98] Karell P, Ahola K, Karstinen T, Valkama J, Brommer JE. Climate change drives microevolution in a wild bird. *Nat Commun*. 2011 Feb;2:208. **PMID: 21343926**

[99] Lerchbaum E, Obermayer-Pietsch BR. Vitamin D and fertility-a systematic review. *Eur J Endocrinol*. 2012 Jan 24. **PMID: 22275473**

[100] Wisborg K, Ingerslev HJ, Henriksen TB. IVF and stillbirth: a prospective follow-up study. *Hum Reprod*. 2010 May;25(5):1312-6. **PMID: 20179321**

[101] Reefhuis J, Honein MA, Schieve LA, Correa A, Hobbs CA, Rasmussen SA; National Birth Defects Prevention Study. Assisted reproductive technology and major structural birth defects in the United States. *Hum Reprod*. 2009 Feb;24(2):360-6. **PMID: 19010807**

[102] Buchala AJ, Pythoud F. Vitamin D and related compounds as plant growth substances. *Physiologia Plantarum*. October 1988. Volume 74, Issue 2, pages 391-396.

[103] Callaway J, Schwab U, Harvima I, Halonen P, Mykkänen O,

Hyvönen P, Järvinen T. Efficacy of dietary hempseed oil in patients with atopic dermatitis. *J Dermatolog Treat.* 2005 Apr;16(2):87-94. **PMID: 16019622**

[104] Schwarz S, Leweling H, Meinck HM. [Alternative and complementary therapies in multiple sclerosis]. *Fortschr Neurol Psychiatr.* 2005 Aug;73(8):451-62. Review. **PMID: 16052439**

[105] Pitcher T, Sergeev IN, Buffenstein R. Vitamin D metabolism in the Damara mole-rat is altered by exposure to sunlight yet mineral metabolism is unaffected. *J Endocrinol.* 1994 Nov;143(2):367-74. **PMID: 7829999**

[106] Cavaleros M, Buffenstein R, Ross FP, Pettifor JM. Vitamin D metabolism in a frugivorous nocturnal mammal, the Egyptian fruit bat (Rousettus aegyptiacus). *Gen Comp Endocrinol.* 2003 Aug;133(1):109-17. **PMID: 12899852**

5. Human D-volution

[107] Holick MF, Chen TC. Vitamin D deficiency: a worldwide problem with health consequences. *Am J Clin Nutr.* 2008 Apr;87(4):1080S-6S. Review. **PMID: 18400738**

[108] Woo DK, Eide MJ. Tanning beds, skin cancer, and vitamin D: An examination of the scientific evidence and public health implications. *Dermatol Ther.* 2010 Jan;23(1):61-71. **PMID: 20136909**

[109] Rise in fraudulent insurance claims. *Financial Times*. March 30, 2010. Retrieved March 3, 2011, from http://v.gd/j0R3WT

[110] Magkos F, Arvaniti F, Zampelas A. Organic food: nutritious food or food for thought? A review of the evidence. *Int J Food Sci Nutr.* 2003 Sep;54(5):357-71. Review. **PMID:**

12907407

[111] Liu H, Prugnolle F, Manica A, Balloux F. A geographically explicit genetic model of worldwide human-settlement history. *Am J Hum Genet.* 2006 Aug;79(2):230-7. **PMID: 16826514**

[112] Lamason RL, Mohideen MA, Mest JR, Wong AC, Norton HL, Aros MC, Jurynec MJ, Mao X, Humphreville VR, Humbert JE, Sinha S, Moore JL, Jagadeeswaran P, Zhao W, Ning G, Makalowska I, McKeigue PM, O'donnell D, Kittles R, Parra EJ, Mangini NJ, Grunwald DJ, Shriver MD, Canfield VA, Cheng KC. SLC24A5, a putative cation exchanger, affects pigmentation in zebrafish and humans. *Science.* 2005 Dec 16;310(5755):1782-6. **PMID: 16357253**

[113] Eiberg H, Troelsen J, Nielsen M, Mikkelsen A, Mengel-From J, Kjaer KW, Hansen L. Blue eye color in humans may be caused by a perfectly associated founder mutation in a regulatory element located within the HERC2 gene inhibiting OCA2 expression. *Hum Genet.* 2008 Mar;123(2):177-87. **PMID: 18172690**

[114] Yuen AW, Jablonski NG. Vitamin D: in the evolution of human skin colour. *Med Hypotheses.* 2010 Jan;74(1):39-44. **PMID: 19717244**

[115] Pearce E, Dunbar R. Latitudinal variation in light levels drives human visual system size. *Biol Lett.* 2012 Feb 23;8(1):90-3. **PMID: 21795263**

[116] Johnson JS, Nobmann ED, Asay E, Lanier AP. Dietary intake of Alaska Native people in two regions and implications for health: the Alaska Native Dietary and Subsistence Food Assessment Project. *Int J Circumpolar Health.* 2009 Apr;68(2):109-22. **PMID: 19517871**

[117] Bjerregaard P, Jørgensen ME, Lumholt P, Mosgaard L,

Borch-Johnsen K; Greenland Population Study. Higher blood pressure among Inuit migrants in Denmark than among the Inuit in Greenland. *J Epidemiol Community Health.* 2002 Apr;56(4):279-84. **PMID: 11896135**

[118] The black woman - with white parents. *The Guardian.* Last updated March 17, 2003. Retrieved March 3, 2011, from http://v.gd/vkN51x

[119] Black and white twins. *Daily Mail.* Last updated March 2, 2006. Retrieved March 3, 2011, from http://v.gd/URFPDq

[120] Findings from the British Crime Survey and police recorded crime (Third edition). Crime in England and Wales 2009/10. Home Office Statistical Bulletin. July 2010. http://v.gd/dsA50p (PDF) see page 1.

[121] Baron-Cohen S. The extreme male brain theory of autism. *Trends Cogn Sci.* 2002 Jun 1;6(6):248-254. **PMID: 12039606**

[122] Nevels RM, Dehon EE, Alexander K, Gontkovsky ST. Psychopharmacology of aggression in children and adolescents with primary neuropsychiatric disorders: a review of current and potentially promising treatment options. *Exp Clin Psychopharmacol.* 2010 Apr;18(2):184-201. **PMID: 20384430**

[123] Social Trends. Office for National Statistics. Last updated July 6, 2010. Retrieved September 24, 2011, from http://v.gd/iQRCRU (PDF) see page 38.

[124] Crawford C, Dearden L, Greaves E. Does when you are born matter? The impact of month of birth on children's cognitive and non-cognitive skills in England. The Institute for Fiscal Studies (IFS Briefing Note BN122). November 2011. http://v.gd/6pfAPI

[125] Hochberg MC. Racial differences in bone strength. *Trans Am Clin Climatol Assoc.* 2007;118:305-15. **PMID: 18528512**

[126] Aloia JF. African Americans, 25-hydroxyvitamin D, and osteoporosis: a paradox. *Am J Clin Nutr.* 2008 Aug;88(2):545S-550S. Review. **PMID: 18689399**

[127] Blacks Are Better Athletes. *The New York Times.* May 28, 1989. Retrieved March 3, 2011, from http://v.gd/xNo9IW

6. Cholesterol & Heart Disease

[128] Duff GL, McMillian GC. Pathology of atherosclerosis. *Am J Med.* 1951 Jul;11(1):92-108. **PMID: 14837929**

[129] Thompson GR, Packard CJ, Stone NJ. Goals of statin therapy: three viewpoints. *Curr Atheroscler Rep.* 2002 Jan;4(1):26-33. Review. **PMID: 11772419**

[130] Clarkson S, Newburgh LH. The relationship between atherosclerosis and ingested cholesterol in the rabbit. *J Exp Med.* 1926 Apr 30;43(5):595-612. **PMID: 19869147**

[131] Kroon AA, Stalenhoef AF. LDL-cholesterol lowering and atherosclerosis--clinical benefit and possible mechanisms: an update. *Neth J Med.* 1997 Jul;51(1):16-27. Review. **PMID: 9260486**

[132] Statin-fortified drinking water? BBC News. Last updated August 1, 2004. Retrieved March 18, 2011, from http://v.gd/1fAxbW

[133] Kim JM, Stewart R, Shin IS, Yoon JS. Low cholesterol, cognitive function and Alzheimer s disease in a community population with cognitive impairment. *J Nutr Health Aging.* 2002;6(5):320-3. **PMID: 12474022**

[134] High cholesterol level (hypercholesterolaemia). NetDoctor. Last updated July 4, 2008. Retrieved March 18, 2011, from http://v.gd/kGQof8

[135] Tall AR, Yvan-Charvet L, Wang N. The failure of torcetrapib: was it the molecule or the mechanism? *Arterioscler Thromb Vasc Biol.* 2007 Feb;27(2):257-60. **PMID: 17229967**

[136] Ridker PM, Danielson E, Fonseca FA, Genest J, Gotto AM Jr, Kastelein JJ, Koenig W, Libby P, Lorenzatti AJ, MacFadyen JG, Nordestgaard BG, Shepherd J, Willerson JT, Glynn RJ; JUPITER Study Group. Rosuvastatin to prevent vascular events in men and women with elevated C-reactive protein. *N Engl J Med.* 2008 Nov 20;359(21):2195-207. **PMID: 18997196**

[137] Grimes DS. Are statins analogues of vitamin D? *Lancet.* 2006 Jul 1;368(9529):83-6. Review. **PMID: 16815382**

[138] Schwartz JB. Effects of vitamin D supplementation in atorvastatin-treated patients: a new drug interaction with an unexpected consequence. *Clin Pharmacol Ther.* 2009 Feb;85(2):198-203. **PMID: 18754003**

[139] Suzuki Y, Ichiyama T, Ohsaki A, Hasegawa S, Shiraishi M, Furukawa S. Anti-inflammatory effect of 1alpha,25-dihydroxyvitamin D(3) in human coronary arterial endothelial cells: Implication for the treatment of Kawasaki disease. *J Steroid Biochem Mol Biol.* 2009 Jan;113(1-2):134-8. **PMID: 19138739**

[140] Rejnmark L, Vestergaard P, Heickendorff L, Mosekilde L. Simvastatin does not affect vitamin d status, but low vitamin d levels are associated with dyslipidemia: results from a randomised, controlled trial. *Int J Endocrinol.* 2010;2010:957174. **PMID: 20016680**

[141] Prospective Studies Collaboration, Lewington S, Whitlock G, Clarke R, Sherliker P, Emberson J, Halsey J, Qizilbash N, Peto R, Collins R. Blood cholesterol and vascular mortality by age, sex, and blood pressure: a meta-analysis of individual data from 61 prospective studies with 55,000 vascular deaths. *Lancet*. 2007 Dec 1;370(9602):1829-39. Review. Erratum in: *Lancet*. 2008 Jul 26;372(9635):292. **PMID: 18061058**

[142] Schneider EB, Efron DT, MacKenzie EJ, Rivara FP, Nathens AB, Jurkovich GJ. Premorbid statin use is associated with improved survival and functional outcomes in older head-injured individuals. *J Trauma*. 2011 Oct;71(4):815-9. **PMID: 21986733**

[143] Marcella SW, David A, Ohman-Strickland PA, Carson J, Rhoads GG. Statin use and fatal prostate cancer: A matched case-control study. *Cancer*. 2011 Dec 16. **PMID: 22180145**

[144] Kalaras MD, Beelman RB. Vitamin D2 Enrichment In Fresh Mushrooms Using Pulsed UV Light. Penn State University. Retrieved March 18, 2011, from http://v.gd/A8ycb5

[145] Pugh PJ, Morris PD, Hall J, Malkin CJ, Asif S, Jones RD, Channer KS, Jones TH. High prevalence of low testosterone levels in men with coronary heart disease and an association with hypertension and obesity - The South Yorkshire study. *Endocrine Abstracts*. 2003, 5 P225 http://v.gd/PHULfU

[146] Traish AM, Saad F, Feeley RJ, Guay A. The dark side of testosterone deficiency: III. Cardiovascular disease. *J Androl*. 2009 Sep-Oct;30(5):477-94. Review. **PMID: 19342698**

[147] Corona G, Boddi V, Balercia G, Rastrelli G, De Vita G, Sforza A, Forti G, Mannucci E, Maggi M. The Effect of statin therapy on testosterone levels in subjects consulting

for erectile dysfunction. *J Sex Med*. 2010 Apr;7(4 Pt 1):1547-56. **PMID: 20141585**

[148] Walsh BW, Schiff I, Rosner B, Greenberg L, Ravnikar V, Sacks FM. Effects of postmenopausal estrogen replacement on the concentrations and metabolism of plasma lipoproteins. *N Engl J Med*. 1991 Oct 24;325(17):1196-204. **PMID: 1922206**

[149] The Cholesterol Myth exposed - Dr Malcolm Kendrick speaks about World Health Organisation data gathered in their MONI-CA study. MONItoring Trends in CArdiovascular Disease. Video uploaded June 7, 2007. Retrieved March 18, 2011, from http://v.gd/fmFrrk

[150] Lüthold S, Berneis K, Bady P, Müller B. Effects of infectious disease on plasma lipids and their diagnostic significance in critical illness. *Eur J Clin Invest*. 2007 Jul;37(7):573-9. **PMID: 17576209**

[151] Hanna EZ, Chou SP, Grant BF. The relationship between drinking and heart disease morbidity in the United States: results from the National Health Interview Survey. *Alcohol Clin Exp Res*. 1997 Feb;21(1):111-8. **PMID: 9046382**

[152] Gettler JF. Hypocholesterolemia in substance abusers. *South Med J*. 1991 Jul;84(7):937. **PMID: 2068650**

[153] Laposata EA. Cocaine-induced heart disease: mechanisms and pathology. *J Thorac Imaging*. 1991 Jan;6(1):68-75. **PMID: 1671228**

[154] Kawahara T, Nishikawa M, Furusawa T, Inazu T, Suzuki G. Effect of atorvastatin and etidronate combination therapy on regression of aortic atherosclerotic plaques evaluated by magnetic resonance imaging. *J Atheroscler Thromb*. 2011;18(5):384-95. **PMID: 21282896**

[155] Tsouli SG, Kiortsis DN, Argyropoulou MI, Mikhailidis DP, Elisaf MS. Pathogenesis, detection and treatment of Achilles tendon xanthomas. *Eur J Clin Invest*. 2005 Apr;35(4):236-44. Review. **PMID: 15816992**

[156] Emerging Risk Factors Collaboration, Di Angelantonio E, Sarwar N, Perry P, Kaptoge S, Ray KK, Thompson A, Wood AM, Lewington S, Sattar N, Packard CJ, Collins R, Thompson SG, Danesh J. Major lipids, apolipoproteins, and risk of vascular disease. *JAMA*. 2009 Nov 11;302(18):1993-2000. **PMID: 19903920**

[157] Lamarche B, Tchernof A, Moorjani S, Cantin B, Dagenais GR, Lupien PJ, Després JP. Small, dense low-density lipoprotein particles as a predictor of the risk of ischemic heart disease in men. Prospective results from the Québec Cardiovascular Study. *Circulation*. 1997 Jan 7;95(1):69-75. **PMID: 8994419**

[158] McNamara JR, Jenner JL, Li Z, Wilson PW, Schaefer EJ. Change in LDL particle size is associated with change in plasma triglyceride concentration. *Arterioscler Thromb*. 1992 Nov;12(11):1284-90. **PMID: 1420088**

[159] Vitamin D increased my cholesterol. The Heart Scan Blog. October 1, 2009. Retrieved March 18, 2011, from http://v.gd/lsqbXx

[160] Shab-Bidar S, Neyestani TR, Djazayery A, Eshraghian MR, Houshiarrad A, Gharavi A, Kalayi A, Shariatzadeh N, Zahedirad M, Khalaji N, Haidari H. Regular consumption of vitamin D-fortified yogurt drink (Doogh) improved endothelial biomarkers in subjects with type 2 diabetes: a randomized double-blind clinical trial. *BMC Med*. 2011 Nov 24;9:125. **PMID: 22114787**

[161] Kaddurah-Daouk R, Baillie RA, Zhu H, Zeng ZB, Wiest

MM, Nguyen UT, Wojnoonski K, Watkins SM, Trupp M, Krauss RM. Enteric microbiome metabolites correlate with response to simvastatin treatment. *PLoS One.* 2011;6(10):e25482. **PMID: 22022402**

[162] Silaste ML, Alfthan G, Aro A, Kesäniemi YA, Hörkkö S. Tomato juice decreases LDL cholesterol levels and increases LDL resistance to oxidation. *Br J Nutr.* 2007 Dec;98(6):1251-8. **PMID: 17617941**

[163] Pilz S, Tomaschitz A, Ritz E, Pieber TR; Medscape. Vitamin D status and arterial hypertension: a systematic review. *Nat Rev Cardiol.* 2009 Oct;6(10):621-30. **PMID: 19687790**

[164] Fiscella K, Winters P, Tancredi D, Franks P. Racial Disparity in Blood Pressure: is Vitamin D a Factor? *J Gen Intern Med.* 2011 Oct;26(10):1105-11. **PMID: 21509604**

7. HIV/AIDS

[165] Mueller NJ, Fux CA, Ledergerber B, Elzi L, Schmid P, Dang T, Magenta L, Calmy A, Vergopoulos A, Bischoff-Ferrari HA; Swiss HIV Cohort Study. High prevalence of severe vitamin D deficiency in combined antiretroviral therapy-naive and successfully treated Swiss HIV patients. *AIDS.* 2010 May 15;24(8):1127-34. **PMID: 20168200**

[166] Ross AC, Judd S, Kumari M, Hileman C, Storer N, Labbato D, Tangpricha V, McComsey GA. Vitamin D is linked to carotid intima-media thickness and immune reconstitution in HIV-positive individuals. *Antivir Ther.* 2011;16(4):555-63. **PMID: 21685543**

[167] Viard JP, Souberbielle JC, Kirk O, Reekie J, Knysz B, Losso M, Gatell J, Pedersen C, Bogner JR, Lundgren JD, Mocroft A; for the EuroSIDA Study Group. Vitamin D and clinical disease progression in HIV infection: results from the

EuroSIDA study. *AIDS*. 2011 Jun 19;25(10):1305-15. **PMID: 21522006**

[168] Centers for Disease Control and Prevention (CDC). A cluster of Kaposi's sarcoma and Pneumocystis carinii pneumonia among homosexual male residents of Los Angeles and Orange Counties, California. *MMWR Morb Mortal Wkly Rep*. 1982 Jun 18;31(23):305-7. **PMID: 6811844**

[169] Sanford D. Back to a Future: One Man's AIDS Tale Shows How Quickly Epidemic Has Turned. *Oncologist*. 1997;2(2):115-120. **PMID: 10388039**

[170] Centers for Disease Control and Prevention (CDC). Opportunistic infections and Kaposi's sarcoma among Haitians in the United States. *MMWR Morb Mortal Wkly Rep*. 1982 Jul 9;31(26):353-4, 360-1. **PMID: 6811853**

[171] U.S. Announces 3 AIDS Discoveries. *Toledo Blade*. April 24, 1984. Retrieved May 5, 2011, from http://v.gd/bzNGSL

[172] Barré-Sinoussi F, Chermann JC, Rey F, Nugeyre MT, Chamaret S, Gruest J, Dauguet C, Axler-Blin C, Vézinet-Brun F, Rouzioux C, Rozenbaum W, Montagnier L. Isolation of a T-lymphotropic retrovirus from a patient at risk for acquired immune deficiency syndrome (AIDS). *Science*. 1983 May 20;220(4599):868-71. **PMID: 6189183**

[173] Gallo RC. A reflection on HIV/AIDS research after 25 years. *Retrovirology*. 2006 Oct 20;3:72. **PMID: 17054781**

[174] Virology and antibodies. British Liver Trust. Retrieved May 5, 2011, from http://v.gd/Bo7EY1

[175] Shenton J. Chapter 14: Does HIV exist? *Positively False: Exposing the Myths Around HIV and AIDS*. I.B. Tauris. December 31, 1998. ISBN-13: 1-86064-333-7. (Out of

print)

[176] How long does it take to go from HIV infection to a diagnosis of AIDS? Living with HIV/AIDS. Centers for Disease Control and Prevention (CDC). Last updated June 21, 2007. Retrieved May 5, 2011, from http://v.gd/Be1Ndh

[177] Kwok S, Higuchi R. Avoiding false positives with PCR. *Nature.* 1989 May 18;339(6221):237-8. Erratum in: *Nature* 1989 Jun 8;339(6224):490. **PMID: 2716852**

[178] Mullis foreword from Peter Duesberg's *Inventing the AIDS Virus.* Regnery Publishing. February 1996. ISBN-13: 978-0895263995. Retrieved May 5, 2011, from http://v.gd/Tn7BT8

[179] Unedited Michael Verney-Elliot interview from "The AIDS Catch" with Professor Luc Montagnier, filmed at The Pasteur Institute, Paris. 1990. Retrieved May 5, 2011, from http://v.gd/Q0VChM (video)

[180] Broder S. The development of antiretroviral therapy and its impact on the HIV-1/AIDS pandemic. *Antiviral Res.* 2010 Jan;85(1):1-18. Review. **PMID: 20018391**

[181] HIV=AIDS: Fact or Fraud? 1997. Retrieved May 5, 2011, from http://v.gd/ooJM9Z (video) see 1h:05m:44s to 1h:06m:35s.

[182] Fischl MA, Parker CB, Pettinelli C, Wulfsohn M, Hirsch MS, Collier AC, Antoniskis D, Ho M, Richman DD, Fuchs E, et al. A randomized controlled trial of a reduced daily dose of zidovudine in patients with the acquired immunodeficiency syndrome. The AIDS Clinical Trials Group. *N Engl J Med.* 1990 Oct 11;323(15):1009-14. **PMID: 1977079**

[183] Fox J, Peters B, Prakash M, Arribas J, Hill A,

Moecklinghoff C. Improvement in vitamin D deficiency following antiretroviral regime change: Results from the MONET trial. *AIDS Res Hum Retroviruses*. 2011 Jan;27(1):29-34. **PMID: 20854196**

[184] Munro CA, Hube B. Anti-fungal therapy at the HAART of viral therapy. *Trends Microbiol*. 2002 Apr;10(4):173-7. **PMID: 11912023**

[185] Gombart AF, Borregaard N, Koeffler HP. Human cathelicidin antimicrobial peptide (CAMP) gene is a direct target of the vitamin D receptor and is strongly up-regulated in myeloid cells by 1,25-dihydroxyvitamin D3. *FASEB J*. 2005 Jul;19(9):1067-77. **PMID: 15985530**

[186] Murphy JT, Mueller GE, Whitman S. Redefining the growth of the heterosexual HIV/AIDS epidemic in Chicago. *J Acquir Immune Defic Syndr Hum Retrovirol*. 1997 Oct 1;16(2):122-6. **PMID: 9358107**

[187] *HIV/AIDS Programme Highlights 2008-2009*. World Health Organisation (WHO). 2010. ISBN: 978-9241599450. Retrieved May 5, 2011, from http://v.gd/lezVfp (PDF) see page 6.

[188] Swanson MD, Winter HC, Goldstein IJ, Markovitz DM. A lectin isolated from bananas is a potent inhibitor of HIV replication. *J Biol Chem*. 2010 Mar 19;285(12):8646-55. **PMID: 20080975**

[189] Gavrovic-Jankulovic M, Poulsen K, Brckalo T, Bobic S, Lindner B, Petersen A. A novel recombinantly produced banana lectin isoform is a valuable tool for glycoproteomics and a potent modulator of the proliferation response in CD3+, CD4+, and CD8+ populations of human PBMCs. *Int J Biochem Cell Biol*. 2008;40(5):929-41. **PMID: 18083059**

[190] Yamamoto N, Ushijima N, Koga Y. Immunotherapy of

HIV-infected patients with Gc protein-derived macrophage activating factor (GcMAF). *J Med Virol*. 2009 Jan;81(1):16-26. **PMID: 19031451**

[191] Matteuzzi M. Endogenous retroviruses as confounding factors in the pathogenesis of AIDS. University of Florence. 2010. Retrieved May 5, 2011, from http://v.gd/nT6YOd (PDF)

[192] Did the Green Monkey Start AIDS? HIV InSite. University of California, San Francisco. Retrieved May 5, 2011, from http://v.gd/v94kuC (obsolete as of January 28, 2012)

[193] Koliadin V. What causes a positive test for HIV-antibodies? *Continuum*. April 1998. Retrieved May 5, 2011, from http://v.gd/66Pnio

[194] Lance T. GRID = Gay-Related Intestinal Dysbiosis? Explaining HIV/AIDS Paradoxes in Terms of Intestinal Dysbiosis. February 2008. Retrieved May 5, 2011, from http://v.gd/ND9GLP (PDF)

[195] Karim SS, Ramjee G. Anal sex and HIV transmission in women. *Am J Public Health*. 1998 Aug;88(8):1265-6. **PMID: 9702169**

[196] Wu S, Liao AP, Xia Y, Li YC, Li JD, Sartor RB, Sun J. Vitamin D receptor negatively regulates bacterial-stimulated NF-kappaB activity in intestine. *Am J Pathol*. 2010 Aug;177(2):686-97. **PMID: 20566739**

[197] Adejumo A, Olabige O, Sivapalan V. Fatal dual infection with Salmonella and Mycobacterium avium complex infection in a patient with advanced acquired immunodeficiency syndrome: a case report. *Cases J*. 2009 Sep 11;2:6773. **PMID: 20181177**

[198] Amid the murk of 'gut flora,' vitamin D receptor emerges as

a key player. PhysOrg.com. July 7, 2010. Retrieved May 5, 2011, from http://v.gd/MOfUYi

[199] Chin'ombe N, Bourn WR, Williamson AL, Shephard EG. Oral vaccination with a recombinant Salmonella vaccine vector provokes systemic HIV-1 subtype C Gag-specific CD4+ Th1 and Th2 cell immune responses in mice. *Virol J.* 2009 Jun 25;6:87. **PMID: 19555490**

[200] Kariuki S, Revathi G, Kariuki N, Kiiru J, Mwituria J, Muyodi J, Githinji JW, Kagendo D, Munyalo A, Hart CA. Invasive multidrug-resistant non-typhoidal Salmonella infections in Africa: zoonotic or anthroponotic transmission? *J Med Microbiol.* 2006 May;55(Pt 5):585-91. **PMID: 16585646**

[201] Schleithoff SS, Zittermann A, Tenderich G, Berthold HK, Stehle P, Koerfer R. Vitamin D supplementation improves cytokine profiles in patients with congestive heart failure: a double-blind, randomized, placebo-controlled trial. *Am J Clin Nutr.* 2006 Apr;83(4):754-9. **PMID: 16600924**

[202] Clerici M, Gori A, Rizzardini G, Richter C, van den Ende I, van't Land B, Georgiou N, Knol J, Garssen J, Lange J. Nutritional Intervention with NR100157 Restores Gut Microbiota in HIV-1-infected Adults Not on HAART and Reduces Systemic Immune Activation. 18th Conference *on Retroviruses and Opportunistic Infections.* February 27 - March 2, 2011. http://v.gd/C1MOfk

[203] Herzlich BC, Schiano TD. Reversal of apparent AIDS dementia complex following treatment with vitamin B12. *J Intern Med.* 1993 Jun;233(6):495-7. **PMID: 8501420**

[204] Norberg B. Turn of tide for oral vitamin B12 treatment. *J Intern Med.* 1999 Sep;246(3):237-8. **PMID: 10475990**

[205] Guéant JL, Safi A, Aimone-Gastin I, Rabesona H,

Bronowicki JP, Plénat F, Bigard MA, Haertlé T. Autoantibodies in pernicious anemia type I patients recognize sequence 251-256 in human intrinsic factor. *Proc Assoc Am Physicians*. 1997 Sep;109(5):462-9. **PMID: 9285945**

[206] Rock Babylon. The Sleaze. September 7, 2001. Retrieved January 7, 2012, from http://v.gd/FVhHMZ

[207] Ozzy Osbourne 'was told he could be HIV positive by doctors'. *The Telegraph*. October 5, 2009. Retrieved May 5, 2011, from http://v.gd/FxeSmf

[208] Tiwari A, Moghal M, Meleagros L. Life threatening abdominal complications following cocaine abuse. *J R Soc Med*. 2006 Feb;99(2):51-2. **PMID: 16449766**

[209] The' TG, Young M, Rosser S. In-utero cocaine exposure and neonatal intestinal perforation: a case report. *J Natl Med Assoc*. 1995 Dec;87(12):889-91. **PMID: 8558622**

[210] Duesberg P, Koehnlein C, Rasnick D. The chemical bases of the various AIDS epidemics: recreational drugs, anti-viral chemotherapy and malnutrition. *J Biosci*. 2003 Jun;28(4):383-412. **PMID: 12799487**

[211] Smith TC, Novella SP. HIV denial in the Internet era. *PLoS Med*. 2007 Aug;4(8):e256. **PMID: 17713982**

[212] Papadopulos-Eleopulos E, Turner VF, Papadimitriou J, Page B, Causer D, Alfonso H, Mhlongo S, Miller T, Maniotis A, Fiala C. A critique of the Montagnier evidence for the HIV/AIDS hypothesis. *Med Hypotheses*. 2004;63(4):597-601. **PMID: 15325002**

[213] Mac Kenzie WR, Davis JP, Peterson DE, Hibbard AJ, Becker G, Zarvan BS. Multiple false-positive serologic tests for HIV, HTLV-1, and hepatitis C following influenza

vaccination, 1991. *JAMA*. 1992 Aug 26;268(8):1015-7. **PMID: 1501307**

[214] Did Luc Montagnier Discover HIV? Djamel Tahi Interview[s] Luc Montagnier. *Continuum*. Winter 1997. Retrieved May 6, 2011, from http://v.gd/Md1KmM

[215] Is HIV the cause of AIDS? An interview [conducted by Christine Johnson] with Eleni Papadopulos-Eleopulos. *Continuum*. Autumn 1997. Retrieved May 6, 2011, from http://v.gd/IFC7dL

[216] Lieberman J. Defying death--HIV mutation to evade cytotoxic T lymphocytes. *N Engl J Med*. 2002 Oct 10;347(15):1203-4. Review. **PMID: 12374884**

[217] *Report of the Tribunal of Inquiry into the Infection with HIV and Hepatitis C of Persons with Haemophilia and Related Matters*. Government of Ireland. 2002. ISBN: 0-7557-1274-9. Retrieved May 6, 2011, from http://v.gd/0CsJRc (PDF)

[218] Fabri M, Stenger S, Shin DM, Yuk JM, Liu PT, Realegeno S, Lee HM, Krutzik SR, Schenk M, Sieling PA, Teles R, Montoya D, Iyer SS, Bruns H, Lewinsohn DM, Hollis BW, Hewison M, Adams JS, Steinmeyer A, Zügel U, Cheng G, Jo EK, Bloom BR, Modlin RL. Vitamin D is required for IFN-gamma-mediated antimicrobial activity of human macrophages. *Sci Transl Med*. 2011 Oct 12;3(104):104ra102. **PMID: 21998409**

[219] Resnick L, Veren K, Salahuddin SZ, Tondreau S, Markham PD. Stability and inactivation of HTLV-III/LAV under clinical and laboratory environments. *JAMA*. 1986 Apr 11;255(14):1887-91. **PMID: 2419594**

[220] Bayer Exposed (HIV Contaminated Vaccine). MSNBC. Video uploaded November 2, 2006. Retrieved May 6, 2011, from http://v.gd/2yYwu8

[221] Wallny TA, Scholz DT, Oldenburg J, Nicolay C, Ezziddin S, Pennekamp PH, Stoffel-Wagner B, Kraft CN. Osteoporosis in haemophilia - an underestimated comorbidity? *Haemophilia.* 2007 Jan;13(1):79-84. **PMID: 17212729**

[222] Welt SI, Graham JB, Kossove DB, Kirkman HN. Vitamin D-resistant rickets and hemophilia A--lack of close linkage on the X chromosome. *Am J Hum Genet.* 1973 Jan;25(1):105-7. **PMID: 4346240**

[223] The plight of Romania's HIV orphans. BBC News. Last updated December 22, 2009. Retrieved May 6, 2011, from http://v.gd/fQ45HC

[224] Brass Eye. Series 2, Episode 1: Paedophillia. Channel 4. Aired July 26, 2001. Retrieved May 6, 2011, from http://v.gd/FDbHcc see 9m:13s to 9m:26s.

[225] Crum-Cianflone N, Roediger MP, Eberly L, Headd M, Marconi V, Ganesan A, Weintrob A, Barthel RV, Fraser S, Agan BK; Infectious Disease Clinical Research Program HIV Working Group. Increasing rates of obesity among HIV-infected persons during the HIV epidemic. *PLoS One.* 2010 Apr 9;5(4):e10106. **PMID: 20419086**

[226] Matemo D, Kinuthia J, John F, Chung M, Farquhar C, John-Stewart G, Kiarie J. Indeterminate rapid HIV-1 test results among antenatal and postnatal mothers. *Int J STD AIDS.* 2009 Nov;20(11):790-2. **PMID: 19875832**

[227] Mehta S, Hunter DJ, Mugusi FM, Spiegelman D, Manji KP, Giovannucci EL, Hertzmark E, Msamanga GI, Fawzi WW. Perinatal outcomes, including mother-to-child transmission of HIV, and child mortality and their association with maternal vitamin D status in Tanzania. *J Infect Dis.* 2009 Oct 1;200(7):1022-30. **PMID: 19673647**

[228] Mestecky J, Ogra PL, McGhee JR, Lambrecht BN, Strober

W. *Mucosal Immunology*. Academic Press; 3ʳᵈ edition. February 2, 2005. ISBN-13: 978-0124915435. See page 312.

[229] Adachi A, Kobayashi T. Identification of vitamin D3 and 7-dehydrocholesterol in cow's milk by gas chromatography-mass spectrometry and their quantitation by high-performance liquid chromatography. *J Nutr Sci Vitaminol (Tokyo)*. 1979;25(2):67-78. **PMID: 225459**

[230] Christine Maggiore and Eliza Jane Scovill: Living and dying with HIV/AIDS denialism. Science-Based Medicine. January 5, 2009. Retrieved May 6, 2011, from http://v.gd/URzW1K

[231] Modan B, Goldschmidt R, Rubinstein E, Vonsover A, Zinn M, Golan R, Chetrit A, Gottlieb-Stematzky T. Prevalence of HIV antibodies in transsexual and female prostitutes. *Am J Public Health*. 1992 Apr;82(4):590-2. **PMID: 1546782**

[232] Nadja Benaissa - Criminal or Victim? HEAL London. Last updated December 2, 2010. Retrieved May 6, 2011, from http://v.gd/YSrYFA

[233] HIV among African Americans - Fact sheet. Centers for Disease Control and Prevention (CDC). September 2010. Retrieved May 6, 2011, from http://v.gd/jfuR78

[234] HIV/AIDS population aging. *Chicago Tribune*. September 24, 2011. Retrieved September 30, 2011, from http://t.co/Ci9Hvq15

[235] NAC spearheads HIV and AIDS work-place programmes. National AIDS Council of Zimbabwe. July 21, 2011. Retrieved January 7, 2012, from http://v.gd/fvy1vX

[236] Yang JH, Lee YM, Bae SG, Jacobs DR Jr, Lee DH. Associations between organochlorine pesticides and vitamin

D deficiency in the U.S. population. *PLoS One.* 2012;7(1):e30093. **PMID: 22295072**

[237] What Are the AIDS Defining Illnesses? About.com. Last updated July 20, 2009. Retrieved January 28, 2012, from http://v.gd/cQJEPM

[238] Nnoaham KE, Clarke A. Low serum vitamin D levels and tuberculosis: a systematic review and meta-analysis. *Int J Epidemiol.* 2008 Feb;37(1):113-9. Review. **PMID: 18245055**

[239] Garfein RS, Lozada R, Liu L, Laniado-Laborin R, Rodwell TC, Deiss R, Alvelais J, Catanzaro A, Chiles PG, Strathdee SA. High prevalence of latent tuberculosis infection among injection drug users in Tijuana, Mexico. *Int J Tuberc Lung Dis.* 2009 May;13(5):626-32. **PMID: 19383197**

[240] Schwenk A, Macallan DC. Tuberculosis, malnutrition and wasting. *Curr Opin Clin Nutr Metab Care.* 2000 Jul;3(4):285-91. Review. **PMID: 10929675**

[241] Finkel TH, Banda NK. Indirect mechanisms of HIV pathogenesis: how does HIV kill T cells? *Curr Opin Immunol.* 1994 Aug;6(4):605-15. Review. **PMID: 7946050**

[242] Ramirez JA, Srinath L, Ahkee S, Huang AK, Raff MJ. HIV-negative "AIDS" in Kentucky: a case of idiopathic CD4+ lymphopenia and cryptococcal meningitis. *South Med J.* 1994 Jul;87(7):751-2. **PMID: 8023211**

[243] Duesberg PH. *Inventing the AIDS Virus*: Appendix B. Regnery Publishing. February 1996. ISBN-13: 978-0895263995. See page 524.

[244] Bone marrow 'cures HIV patient'. BBC News. Last updated November 13, 2008. Retrieved May 6, 2011, from http://v.gd/xoFvLL

[245] Galvani AP, Novembre J. The evolutionary history of the CCR5-Delta32 HIV-resistance mutation. *Microbes Infect.* 2005 Feb;7(2):302-9. Review. **PMID: 15715976**

[246] Nabatov AA, Pollakis G, Linnemann T, Paxton WA, de Baar MP. Statins disrupt CCR5 and RANTES expression levels in CD4(+) T lymphocytes in vitro and preferentially decrease infection of R5 versus X4 HIV-1. *PLoS One.* 2007 May 23;2(5):e470. **PMID: 17520029**

[247] Moore RD, Bartlett JG, Gallant JE. Association between use of HMG CoA reductase inhibitors and mortality in HIV-infected patients. *PLoS One.* 2011;6(7):e21843. **PMID: 21765919**

[248] AIDS truth exposed: Un-cut exclusive footage from *House of Numbers*. Uploaded November 30, 2009. Retrieved May 6, 2011, from http://v.gd/3FcXwL

[249] Montagnier: Still No Denial. Inside *House of Numbers*. Last updated December 3, 2009. Retrieved May 6, 2011, from http://v.gd/iLnlyJ

8. Approaching Repletion

[250] Holick MF, Biancuzzo RM, Chen TC, Klein EK, Young A, Bibuld D, Reitz R, Salameh W, Ameri A, Tannenbaum AD. Vitamin D2 is as effective as vitamin D3 in maintaining circulating concentrations of 25-hydroxyvitamin D. *J Clin Endocrinol Metab.* 2008 Mar;93(3):677-81. **PMID: 18089691**

[251] Armas LA, Hollis BW, Heaney RP. Vitamin D2 is much less effective than vitamin D3 in humans. *J Clin Endocrinol Metab.* 2004 Nov;89(11):5387-91. **PMID: 15531486**

[252] How vitamin D is made from sheep wool. Vitamin D Wiki.

Last updated October 2011. Retrieved January 28, 2012, from http://v.gd/PhsatI

[253] Restless Legs Syndrome (see sidebar). NHS. Last reviewed November 6, 2009. Retrieved January 28, 2011, from http://v.gd/oXyWLQ

[254] Smith DC, Johnson CS, Freeman CC, Muindi J, Wilson JW, Trump DL. A Phase I trial of calcitriol (1,25-dihydroxycholecalciferol) in patients with advanced malignancy. *Clin Cancer Res*. 1999 Jun;5(6):1339-45. **PMID: 10389917**

[255] Brown AJ. Therapeutic uses of vitamin D analogues. *Am J Kidney Dis*. 2001 Nov;38(5 Suppl 5):S3-S19. Review. **PMID: 11689383**

[256] Tiwari A. Elocalcitol, a vitamin D3 analog for the potential treatment of benign prostatic hyperplasia, overactive bladder and male infertility. *IDrugs*. 2009 Jun;12(6):381-93. **PMID: 19517319**

[257] Climate change emails between scientists reveal flaws in peer review. *The Guardian*. Last updated February 16, 2012. Retrieved July 21, 2012, from http://v.gd/50XdDt

[258] Vitamin D: The Test. Lab Tests Online. Last updated December 21, 2011. Retrieved January 28, 2011, from http://v.gd/WPCO7W

[259] NOW Recalls Calcium & Magnesium Softgels Due to Excessive Amounts of Vitamin D3. Natural Grocers. May 26, 2011. Retrieved January 28, 2012, from http://v.gd/XIlQlD

[260] Tzotzas T, Papadopoulou FG, Tziomalos K, Karras S, Gastaris K, Perros P, Krassas GE. Rising serum 25-hydroxy-vitamin D levels after weight loss in obese women

correlate with improvement in insulin resistance. *J Clin Endocrinol Metab.* 2010 Sep;95(9):4251-7. **PMID: 20534751**

[261] Maetani M, Maskarinec G, Franke AA, Cooney RV. Association of leptin, 25-hydroxyvitamin D, and parathyroid hormone in women. *Nutr Cancer.* 2009;61(2):225-31. **PMID: 19235038**

[262] Galgani JE, Greenway FL, Caglayan S, Wong ML, Licinio J, Ravussin E. Leptin replacement prevents weight loss-induced metabolic adaptation in congenital leptin-deficient patients. *J Clin Endocrinol Metab.* 2010 Feb;95(2):851-5. **PMID: 20061423**

[263] Skversky AL, Kumar J, Abramowitz MK, Kaskel FJ, Melamed ML. Association of Glucocorticoid Use and Low 25-Hydroxyvitamin D Levels: Results from the National Health and Nutrition Examination Survey (NHANES): 2001-2006. *J Clin Endocrinol Metab.* 2011 Dec;96(12):3838-45. **PMID: 21956424**

[264] Eckstein C, et al. Vitamin D3 content in commercially available oral supplements. *CMSC-ACTRIMS.* 2010; P. 33-34.

[265] Shah BR, Finberg L. Single-day therapy for nutritional vitamin D-deficiency rickets: a preferred method. *J Pediatr.* 1994 Sep;125(3):487-90. **PMID: 8071764**

[266] Tangpricha V, Turner A, Spina C, Decastro S, Chen TC, Holick MF. Tanning is associated with optimal vitamin D status (serum 25-hydroxyvitamin D concentration) and higher bone mineral density. *Am J Clin Nutr.* 2004 Dec;80(6):1645-9. **PMID: 15585781**

[267] Vitamin D: UV Sensors and Sheer Sunscreen. SkinHealth Technology, LLC. Retrieved June 12, 2011, from

http://v.gd/A9UlaC

[268] Melanoma and Skin of Color. The Skin Cancer Foundation. January 29, 2009. Retrieved June 12, 2011, from http://v.gd/7kNoFR

[269] Reichrath J. Sunlight, skin cancer and vitamin D: What are the conclusions of recent findings that protection against solar ultraviolet (UV) radiation causes 25-hydroxyvitamin D deficiency in solid organ-transplant recipients, xeroderma pigmentosum, and other risk groups? *J Steroid Biochem Mol Biol*. 2007 Mar;103(3-5):664-7. **PMID: 17204418**

[270] Introduction to the Marshall Protocol. The Marshall Protocol Knowledge Base. Last updated January 2, 2012. Retrieved January 28, 2012, from http://v.gd/JxuaJs

[271] Information About Trevor Marshall, Ph.D. Retrieved June 12, 2011, from http://v.gd/xFDjJV

[272] Mechanisms by which bacteria affect levels of vitamin D. The Marshall Protocol Knowledge Base. Last updated January 2, 2012. Retrieved January 28, 2012, from http://v.gd/X4hHcQ

[273] Professor Marshall's recent "discovery". Vitamin D Council News Archive. Last updated October 11, 2011. Retrieved January 28, 2012, from http://v.gd/3dTre2

[274] Insogna KL, Dreyer BE, Mitnick M, Ellison AF, Broadus AE. Enhanced production rate of 1,25-dihydroxyvitamin D in sarcoidosis. *J Clin Endocrinol Metab*. 1988 Jan;66(1):72-5. **PMID: 3335611**

[275] FDA Drug Safety Communication: Safety Review Update of Benicar (olmesartan) and cardiovascular events. U.S. Food and Drug Administration (FDA). Last updated April 14, 2011. Retrieved June 12, 2011, from http://v.gd/5UNNSu

[276] Sipahi I, Debanne SM, Rowland DY, Simon DI, Fang JC. Angiotensin-receptor blockade and risk of cancer: meta-analysis of randomised controlled trials. *Lancet Oncol*. 2010 Jul;11(7):627-36. Review. **PMID: 20542468**

[277] Sponsors and Collaborators: University of Wisconsin, Madison and Merck. Improving the Understanding of the Response to Vitamin D Supplementation. Last updated November 13, 2011. Retrieved January 7, 2012 via ClinicalTrials.gov Identifier: **NCT01465178**

[278] Schlingmann KP, Kaufmann M, Weber S, Irwin A, Goos C, John U, Misselwitz J, Klaus G, Kuwertz-Bröking E, Fehrenbach H, Wingen AM, Güran T, Hoenderop JG, Bindels RJ, Prosser DE, Jones G, Konrad M. Mutations in CYP24A1 and idiopathic infantile hypercalcemia. *N Engl J Med*. 2011 Aug 4;365(5):410-21. **PMID: 21675912**

9. Influenza & Autoimmunity

[279] Reis AF, Hauache OM, Velho G. Vitamin D endocrine system and the genetic susceptibility to diabetes, obesity and vascular disease. A review of evidence. *Diabetes Metab*. 2005 Sep;31(4 Pt 1):318-25. Review. **PMID: 16369193**

[280] Small CL, Shaler CR, McCormick S, Jeyanathan M, Damjanovic D, Brown EG, Arck P, Jordana M, Kaushic C, Ashkar AA, Xing Z. Influenza infection leads to increased susceptibility to subsequent bacterial superinfection by impairing NK cell responses in the lung. *J Immunol*. 2010 Feb 15;184(4):2048-56. **PMID: 20083661**

[281] Urashima M, Segawa T, Okazaki M, Kurihara M, Wada Y, Ida H. Randomized trial of vitamin D supplementation to prevent seasonal influenza A in schoolchildren. *Am J Clin*

Nutr. 2010 May;91(5):1255-60. **PMID: 20219962**

[282] Maclean M, MacGregor SJ, Anderson JG, Woolsey G. Inactivation of bacterial pathogens following exposure to light from a 405-nanometer light-emitting diode array. *Appl Environ Microbiol.* 2009 Apr;75(7):1932-7. **PMID: 19201962**

[283] Douglas RM, Hemilä H, Chalker E, Treacy B. Vitamin C for preventing and treating the common cold. *Cochrane Database Syst Rev.* 2007 Jul 18;(3):CD000980. Review. **PMID: 17636648**

[284] Misra M, Pacaud D, Petryk A, Collett-Solberg PF, Kappy M; Drug and Therapeutics Committee of the Lawson Wilkins Pediatric Endocrine Society. Vitamin D deficiency in children and its management: review of current knowledge and recommendations. *Pediatrics.* 2008 Aug;122(2):398-417. Review. **PMID: 18676559**

[285] Cohen D, Carter P. Conflicts of interest. WHO and the pandemic flu "conspiracies". *BMJ.* 2010 Jun 3;340:c2912. **PMID: 20525679**

[286] Santón A, Cristóbal E, Aparicio M, Royuela A, Villar LM, Alvarez-Cermeño JC. High frequency of co-infection by Epstein-Barr virus types 1 and 2 in patients with multiple sclerosis. *Mult Scler.* 2011 Nov;17(11):1295-300. **PMID: 21757537**

[287] Lang HL, Jacobsen H, Ikemizu S, Andersson C, Harlos K, Madsen L, Hjorth P, Sondergaard L, Svejgaard A, Wucherpfennig K, Stuart DI, Bell JI, Jones EY, Fugger L. A functional and structural basis for TCR cross-reactivity in multiple sclerosis. *Nat Immunol.* 2002 Oct;3(10):940-3. **PMID: 12244309**

[288] Pollock BJ, McKenzie AS, Kemp BE, McPhee DA, D'Apice

AJ. Human monoclonal antibodies to HIV-1: cross-reactions with gag and env products. *Clin Exp Immunol.* 1989 Dec;78(3):323-8. **PMID: 2482145**

[289] Sreeram Ramagopalan Part 2 - Sunlight and Vitamin D: key factors? Video uploaded April 23, 2010. Retrieved July 27, 2010, from http://v.gd/8ZjPG5

[290] Brennan RM, Burrows JM, Bell MJ, Bromham L, Csurhes PA, Lenarczyk A, Sverndal J, Klintenstedt J, Pender MP, Burrows SR. Strains of Epstein-Barr virus infecting multiple sclerosis patients. *Mult Scler.* 2010 Jun;16(6):643-51. **PMID: 20350958**

[291] Rothwell PM, Charlton D. High incidence and prevalence of multiple sclerosis in south east Scotland: evidence of a genetic predisposition. *J Neurol Neurosurg Psychiatry.* 1998 Jun;64(6):730-5. **PMID: 9647300**

[292] Ramagopalan SV, Dyment DA, Cader MZ, Morrison KM, Disanto G, Morahan JM, Berlanga-Taylor AJ, Handel A, De Luca GC, Sadovnick AD, Lepage P, Montpetit A, Ebers GC. Rare variants in the CYP27B1 gene are associated with multiple sclerosis. *Ann Neurol.* 2011 Dec;70(6):881-6. **PMID: 22190362**

[293] Poor health 'due to wet climate'. BBC News. Last updated September 15, 2008. Retrieved July 17, 2011, from http://v.gd/8iQFLV

[294] Glandular Fever. NHS Choices. Last updated January 25, 2011. Retrieved July 18, 2011, from http://v.gd/KF1rO5

[295] Elian M, Nightingale S, Dean G. Multiple sclerosis among United Kingdom-born children of immigrants from the Indian subcontinent, Africa and the West Indies. *J Neurol Neurosurg Psychiatry.* 1990 Oct;53(10):906-11. **PMID: 2266374**

[296] Simpson S Jr, Taylor B, Blizzard L, Ponsonby AL, Pittas F, Tremlett H, Dwyer T, Gies P, van der Mei I. Higher 25-hydroxyvitamin D is associated with lower relapse risk in multiple sclerosis. *Ann Neurol.* 2010 Aug;68(2):193-203. **PMID: 20695012**

[297] DeLorenze GN, Munger KL, Lennette ET, Orentreich N, Vogelman JH, Ascherio A. Epstein-Barr virus and multiple sclerosis: evidence of association from a prospective study with long-term follow-up. *Arch Neurol.* 2006 Jun;63(6):839-44. **PMID: 16606758**

[298] Becklund BR, Severson KS, Vang SV, DeLuca HF. UV radiation suppresses experimental autoimmune encephalomyelitis independent of vitamin D production. *Proc Natl Acad Sci U S A.* 2010 Apr 6;107(14):6418-23. **PMID: 20308557**

[299] Honeyman MC, Stone NL, Falk BA, Nepom G, Harrison LC. Evidence for molecular mimicry between human T cell epitopes in rotavirus and pancreatic islet autoantigens. *J Immunol.* 2010 Feb 15;184(4):2204-10. **PMID: 20083660**

[300] Hyppönen E, Läärä E, Reunanen A, Järvelin MR, Virtanen SM. Intake of vitamin D and risk of type 1 diabetes: a birth-cohort study. *Lancet.* 2001 Nov 3;358(9292):1500-3. **PMID: 11705562**

[301] Kohn LD, Wallace B, Schwartz F, McCall K. Is type 2 diabetes an autoimmune-inflammatory disorder of the innate immune system? *Endocrinology.* 2005 Oct;146(10):4189-91. **PMID: 16166230**

[302] Lim EL, Hollingsworth KG, Aribisala BS, Chen MJ, Mathers JC, Taylor R. Reversal of type 2 diabetes: normalisation of beta cell function in association with decreased pancreas and liver triacylglycerol. *Diabetologia.*

2011 Oct;54(10):2506-14. **PMID: 21656330**

[303] Knekt P, Laaksonen M, Mattila C, Härkänen T, Marniemi J, Heliövaara M, Rissanen H, Montonen J, Reunanen A. Serum vitamin D and subsequent occurrence of type 2 diabetes. *Epidemiology.* 2008 Sep;19(5):666-71. **PMID: 18496468**

[304] American Diabetes Association. Standards of medical care in diabetes--2011. *Diabetes Care.* 2011 Jan;34 Suppl 1:S11-61. **PMID: 21193625**

[305] Harjutsalo V, Sjöberg L, Tuomilehto J. Time trends in the incidence of type 1 diabetes in Finnish children: a cohort study. *Lancet.* 2008 May 24;371(9626):1777-82. **PMID: 18502302**

[306] Traish AM, Saad F, Guay A. The dark side of testosterone deficiency: II. Type 2 diabetes and insulin resistance. *J Androl.* 2009 Jan-Feb;30(1):23-32. Review. **PMID: 18772488**

10. Popping Cancer

[307] Sasieni PD, Shelton J, Ormiston-Smith N, Thomson CS, Silcocks PB. What is the lifetime risk of developing cancer?: the effect of adjusting for multiple primaries. *Br J Cancer.* 2011 Jul 26;105(3):460-5. **PMID: 21772332**

[308] What causes cancer? CancerHelp UK. Cancer Research UK. Last updated January 25, 2012. Retrieved January 29, 2012, from http://v.gd/gZKZGZ

[309] Walboomers JM, Jacobs MV, Manos MM, Bosch FX, Kummer JA, Shah KV, Snijders PJ, Peto J, Meijer CJ, Muñoz N. Human papillomavirus is a necessary cause of invasive cervical cancer worldwide. *J Pathol.* 1999

Sep;189(1):12-9. **PMID: 10451482**

[310] 'I have a brain tumour.' BBC News. Last updated September 12, 2002. Retrieved August 23, 2011, from http://v.gd/GXrywo

[311] Why 5 A DAY? NHS Choices. Last updated December 5, 2011. Retrieved January 29, 2012, from http://v.gd/UZjQ6q

[312] Filip B, Milczarek M, Wietrzyk J, Chodyński M, Kutner A. Antitumor properties of (5E,7E) analogs of vitamin D3. *J Steroid Biochem Mol Biol.* 2010 Jul;121(1-2):399-402. **PMID: 20227499**

[313] Krishnan AV, Trump DL, Johnson CS, Feldman D. The role of vitamin D in cancer prevention and treatment. *Endocrinol Metab Clin North Am.* 2010 Jun;39(2):401-18, table of contents. Review. **PMID: 20511060**

[314] Lappe JM, Travers-Gustafson D, Davies KM, Recker RR, Heaney RP. Vitamin D and calcium supplementation reduces cancer risk: results of a randomized trial. *Am J Clin Nutr.* 2007 Jun;85(6):1586-91. Erratum in: *Am J Clin Nutr.* 2008 Mar;87(3):794. **PMID: 17556697**

[315] Ma Y, Yu WD, Trump DL, Johnson CS. 1,25D3 enhances antitumor activity of gemcitabine and cisplatin in human bladder cancer models. *Cancer.* 2010 Jul 1;116(13):3294-303. **PMID: 20564622**

[316] Breast Cancer Rates by Race and Ethnicity. Centers for Disease Control and Prevention (CDC). Last updated September 28, 2010. Retrieved August 23, 2011, from http://v.gd/ptIU3U

[317] Bowen RL, Duffy SW, Ryan DA, Hart IR, Jones JL. Early onset of breast cancer in a group of British black women. *Br J Cancer.* 2008 Jan 29;98(2):277-81. **PMID: 18182985**

[318] McCormack VA, Mangtani P, Bhakta D, McMichael AJ, dos Santos Silva I. Heterogeneity of breast cancer risk within the South Asian female population in England: a population-based case-control study of first-generation migrants. *Br J Cancer*. 2004 Jan 12;90(1):160-6. **PMID: 14710224**

[319] Aggarwal BB, Kumar A, Bharti AC. Anticancer potential of curcumin: preclinical and clinical studies. *Anticancer Res*. 2003 Jan-Feb;23(1A):363-98. Review. **PMID: 12680238**

[320] Skin Cancer Rates by Race and Ethnicity. Centers for Disease Control and Prevention (CDC). Last updated September 27, 2010. Retrieved August 24, 2011, from http://v.gd/pb5moc

[321] Public advice on suntanning may mean vitamin deficiency risk. *The Independent*. July 5, 2010. Retrieved August 27, 2011, from http://v.gd/kau5yd

[322] Obesity, heavy drinking and 'couch potato' lifestyle fuels 20% rise in cancer among the middle aged. *Daily Mail*. Last updated July 18, 2011. Retrieved August 27, 2011, from http://v.gd/ErJVlV

[323] Stickel F, Schuppan D, Hahn EG, Seitz HK. Cocarcinogenic effects of alcohol in hepatocarcinogenesis. *Gut*. 2002 Jul;51(1):132-9. Review. **PMID: 12077107**

[324] Ahn J, Lim U, Weinstein SJ, Schatzkin A, Hayes RB, Virtamo J, Albanes D. Prediagnostic total and high-density lipoprotein cholesterol and risk of cancer. *Cancer Epidemiol Biomarkers Prev*. 2009 Nov;18(11):2814-21. **PMID: 19887581**

[325] Kim Y, Park SK, Han W, Kim DH, Hong YC, Ha EH, Ahn SH, Noh DY, Kang D, Yoo KY. Serum high-density lipoprotein cholesterol and breast cancer risk by

menopausal status, body mass index, and hormonal receptor in Korea. *Cancer Epidemiol Biomarkers Prev*. 2009 Feb;18(2):508-15. **PMID: 19190159**

[326] Robien K, Cutler GJ, Lazovich D. Vitamin D intake and breast cancer risk in postmenopausal women: the Iowa Women's Health Study. *Cancer Causes Control*. 2007 Sep;18(7):775-82. **PMID: 17549593**

[327] McCallum H. Tasmanian devil facial tumour disease: lessons for conservation biology. *Trends Ecol Evol*. 2008 Nov;23(11):631-7. Review. **PMID: 18715674**

[328] Nowak RM. *Walker's Mammals of the World, Volume 2*. The Johns Hopkins University Press; sixth edition. April 7, 1999. ISBN-13: 978-0801857898. See page 64.

[329] The Last of the Tasmanian Devils (and Other Critters). *Time*. October 6, 2008. Retrieved August 27, 2011, from http://v.gd/EmFlhA

Interview: Prof. Bruce Hollis

[330] Priemel M, von Domarus C, Klatte TO, Kessler S, Schlie J, Meier S, Proksch N, Pastor F, Netter C, Streichert T, Püschel K, Amling M. Bone mineralization defects and vitamin D deficiency: histomorphometric analysis of iliac crest bone biopsies and circulating 25-hydroxyvitamin D in 675 patients. *J Bone Miner Res*. 2010 Feb;25(2):305-12. **PMID: 19594303**

11. A Brighter Future

[331] UV light to combat drug use in public toilets. Austrian Times. May 17, 2010. Retrieved October 7, 2011, from http://v.gd/Bxpl3T

[332] Hess AF, Unger LJ. The cure of infantile rickets by sunlight. *JAMA*. 1921;77(1):39.

[333] Terpstra FG, van 't Wout AB, Schuitemaker H, van Engelenburg FA, Dekkers DW, Verhaar R, de Korte D, Verhoeven AJ. Potential and limitation of UVC irradiation for the inactivation of pathogens in platelet concentrates. *Transfusion*. 2008 Feb;48(2):304-13. **PMID: 18028277**

[334] Reichrath J. *Molecular Mechanisms of Basal Cell and Squamous Cell Carcinomas*. Springer. April 26, 2006. ISBN-13: 978-0387260464. See pages 19-20.

[335] Pair cleared over Jayden Wray death. BBC News. Last updated December 9, 2011. Retrieved February 1, 2012, from http://v.gd/4oRXZD

[336] Hitz MF, Jensen JE. [Potentially beneficial effects of climate changes]. *Ugeskr Laeger*. 2009 Oct 26;171(44):3197-200. **PMID: 19857402**

[337] Blask DE. Melatonin, sleep disturbance and cancer risk. *Sleep Med Rev*. 2009 Aug;13(4):257-64. Review. **PMID: 19095474**

[338] Richard Dawkins on why science is better than myth. BBC Newsnight. Aired September 13, 2011. Retrieved October 8, 2011, from http://v.gd/QfffYs see 3m:19s to 3m:23s.

[339] Warraq I. *Why I Am Not a Muslim*. Prometheus Books; Amazon Kindle Edition. June 30, 2010. ISBN-13: 978-1591020110 (physical). See page 40.

Index

1

2

A

E

G

J

K

Further Information

The Vitamin D Association – vitamindassociation.org

THINCS - The International Network Of Cholesterol Skeptics – thincs.org

HIV/AIDS Skepticism – hivskeptic.wordpress.com

Could It Be B12?: An Epidemic of Misdiagnoses by Sally M. Pacholok and Jeffrey J. Stuart (World Dancer Press, 2nd edition, 2011) – b12awareness.org

Acknowledgements

I would like to thank my family and friends... Some of the content here will be more of a revelation to them. Thanks also to those who kindly agreed to be interviewed, and the doctors who have ensured the well-being of my family.

Additionally, I pay tribute to the wealth of relevant information online, particularly the PubMed database [http://www.ncbi.nlm.nih.gov/pubmed], without which this book would not have even been an idea.

Last, but not least, thanks to everyone who provided any form of interest or encouragement towards this project.